THE LONGEVITY BLUEPRINT

Unlock Your Healthspan

by

Riley Vantor

The Longevity Blueprint: Unlock Your Healthspan: A Practical Guide to Living Longer, Healthier, and More Vibrantly

TABLE OF CONTENTS

Chapter One
INTRODUCTION

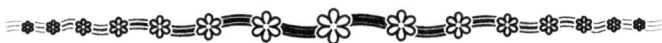

Longevity—the idea of living not just longer, but better—has fascinated humans for centuries. We all have a natural desire to extend our time on this planet, not merely to add years, but to fill those years with health, energy, and purpose. In recent decades, scientific advances have shifted longevity from a mystical dream into a practical, evidence-based pursuit. Unlike the potions and myths of old, today's longevity strategies are rooted in biology, psychology, and lifestyle science.

But living longer is only part of the story. Equally important is sustaining a high quality of life as we age. It's not enough to simply add years; those years must be vibrant, independent, and fulfilling. This book is designed for health-conscious individuals who are ready to take control of their aging journey by adopting strategies that support both lifespan and healthspan—the portion of life spent free from chronic disease and disability.

The path to longevity begins by understanding that aging is not a predetermined curse but a modifiable process. Various factors influence how we age—genes, environment, behavior—and their interplay determines the trajectory of our health. While we can't control our genetic inheritance, emerging research has illuminated how lifestyle choices profoundly affect the aging process. This means the power to shape our future health lies largely in our own hands.

Throughout this book, you'll find guidance that strips away the confusion surrounding longevity trends and fads. There's a flood of information circulating about diets, supplements, and exercise routines promising miraculous results. Here, you'll discover which approaches are backed by science, which are still unproven, and how to tailor concepts to fit your unique needs and circumstances.

What sets this book apart is its practical focus. It isn't enough to know that certain habits might

8

help; you'll be equipped to integrate them into your daily routine in sustainable ways. Longevity is a lifelong journey, and attempts at radical overnight transformations rarely stick. Building a healthier, longer life depends on small but deliberate choices that accumulate over time.

One of the key messages you'll encounter is the holistic nature of aging well. Longevity isn't just about diet or exercise alone. It involves a delicate balance of mental resilience, emotional health, social connection, hormonal balance, quality sleep, and a supportive environment. Ignoring any one of these factors can undermine progress in others. This interconnected approach will be unpacked in detail in the chapters ahead.

It's also important to recognize that aging is an individual experience. What works for one person may not be ideal for another, whether due to genetics, lifestyle history, or personal preferences. That's why this book encourages a personalized approach. By understanding the core principles and science behind healthy aging, you'll be empowered to make informed decisions that align with your body, mind, and goals.

One of the transformative aspects of modern longevity science is the emphasis on prevention rather than just treatment. Historically, much of medicine has focused on managing disease after it occurs. But longevity research urges a shift toward preserving function and delaying the onset of age-related diseases well before symptoms arise.

This preventive mindset opens up exciting possibilities. It means adopting lifestyle habits not purely for short-term benefit but with an eye on how they accumulate to protect health decades down the road. It invites questions like: How do the foods I eat today influence my risk of heart disease 20 years from now? How does my daily stress impact my cognitive function as I reach my 70s and 80s? The answers shape lifelong strategies, reminding us that each choice matters.

Another compelling reason to invest in longevity strategies is the broader impact beyond just individual health. Longer, healthier lives contribute to families, communities, and society in profound ways. Imagine extending not only your years but also the years you can spend actively engaging with loved ones, pursuing passions, and contributing your skills and wisdom.

In the chapters to come, you'll explore the biological forces that drive aging and how to influence them. You'll learn about nutrition plans that reduce inflammation and promote cellular repair. You'll discover the synergistic effects of combining different types of physical activity for lifelong vitality. Mental wellness will be examined as a cornerstone of extended health, including how managing stress and fostering neuroplasticity protect cognitive function.

The science of sleep, often overlooked, emerges as an essential pillar, guiding you to optimize rest for cellular recovery and hormonal balance. Genetics and epigenetics reveal the fascinating dynamic between inherited traits and lifestyle, giving you tools to harness your genetic potential. You'll also explore immune resilience, understanding how a robust defense system shifts the odds toward longevity.

Technology too plays a role, with cutting-edge therapies and innovations expanding the toolkit for healthspan extension—though ethical and accessibility questions remain important. Finally, you'll be invited to embrace the power of social connections and clean environments, areas which are sometimes neglected but have profound effects on well-being and lifespan.

At its core, this book aims to inspire action. Knowledge alone won't extend your life or improve how you feel day to day. The real power lies in applying what you learn, cultivating habits that endure, and adapting as you grow. Most importantly, you'll be encouraged to view longevity not as a restrictive obligation but as a hopeful, empowering journey toward a more vibrant and meaningful life.

The first step might be the hardest—to decide you want to prioritize your future self. But once you take that step, everything else follows. The evidence for longevity practices grows stronger every year, and the opportunity to live a long, healthy life is more within reach than ever before. This introduction sets the stage for a transformative exploration, one that will equip and motivate you every step of the way.

Welcome to a new chapter in your life. One where vitality and wisdom increase with the years, where aging becomes a process of discovery and empowerment rather than decline. Now, let's begin by understanding the fascinating science that underpins the journey toward extended health and lifespan.

Chapter Two
FOUNDATIONS OF LONGEVITY SCIENCE

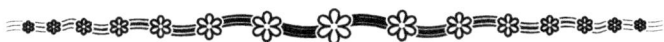

Understanding how and why we age sets the stage for taking control of our healthspan—the period when we live not just longer, but better. Longevity science digs deep into the biological processes that drive aging, revealing that it's not merely about adding years but enhancing vitality through measurable markers like cellular function and systemic resilience. This foundation challenges us to rethink aging as a modifiable journey rather than an inevitable decline. By grounding ourselves in the science behind these mechanisms, we become empowered to make intentional choices that nurture our bodies at their core, inspiring a proactive approach to well-being that's as much about quality as quantity of life.

BIOLOGY BEHIND AGING

Understanding what happens to our bodies at the cellular and molecular levels as we age is key to unlocking the secrets of longevity. Aging isn't just about getting older chronologically—it's about the gradual decline in biological function, the wear and tear that accumulates silently within our cells, tissues, and organs over time. This decline influences everything from how efficiently our body repairs itself to how well our systems remain balanced and resilient. If you're looking to extend not only your lifespan but also your healthspan—the number of years spent in good health—it's essential to grasp the biological forces at work behind the scenes.

At its core, aging is driven by a complex interplay of molecular damage and the body's diminishing ability to respond effectively. Think of it like a finely tuned machine: over the years, tiny parts begin to degrade. Our cells accumulate damage to their DNA, proteins misfold or break down, and energy production within mitochondria—the powerhouses of the cell—slows. While these changes may seem small on their own, their cumulative effect profoundly impacts how our bodies function.

One of the most fundamental biological hallmarks of aging involves genomic instability. DNA damage accrues with every cell division and exposure to environmental stressors like ultraviolet radiation or toxins. Though our bodies have built-in repair systems, their efficiency wanes over time, allowing mutations and errors to accumulate. This gradual erosion of DNA integrity undermines cellular function, increases the risk of diseases, and contributes to the aging phenotype.

Alongside DNA damage, another key player is the shortening of telomeres, those protective caps at the ends of chromosomes. Each time a cell divides, these telomeres shrink, eventually reaching a critical length that triggers cellular senescence—a state where cells stop dividing and enter a kind of biological retirement. Senescent cells aren't merely inert; they secrete inflammatory molecules and other substances that can undermine neighboring cells, fostering a tissue environment rife with chronic, low-grade inflammation, commonly called "inflammaging." This persistent inflammation is a subtle but powerful force that drives many age-related diseases.

Energy metabolism shifts, too. Mitochondrial dysfunction appears early in the aging process and may be considered a central culprit. These organelles specialize in producing ATP, the energy currency of cells, but over time, their efficiency declines, and they release more reactive oxygen species (ROS). These molecules are essentially free radicals, unstable compounds that cause oxidative stress by damaging proteins, lipids, and DNA in cells. The balance between ROS production and antioxidant defenses becomes disrupted, tipping the scale toward damage accumulation. However, emerging research suggests ROS aren't simply harmful; in moderate amounts, they play crucial roles in cellular signaling and adaptation. The trick lies in maintaining that delicate balance.

The accumulation of misfolded or damaged proteins also contributes significantly to aging. Proteostasis—the process cells use to manufacture, fold, and dispose of proteins—deteriorates with time. When proteins clump together, they interfere with normal cellular activities. This is especially evident in neurodegenerative diseases, where protein aggregates can disrupt brain function. But proteostasis is a universal challenge for cells, and impaired protein quality control underlies many age-related functional declines.

Cells themselves don't all age uniformly. Some enter senescence, while others respond by activating repair or recycling systems like autophagy—the cell's way of cleaning out damaged components. Autophagy helps maintain cellular health by breaking down dysfunctional organelles and proteins, thus preventing their harmful accumulation. Unfortunately, autophagy efficiency decreases with age, leaving more cellular waste to accumulate and impair function. Encouragingly, lifestyle interventions such as exercise and caloric restriction have been shown to boost autophagy, promoting cellular rejuvenation.

At the tissue level, aging manifests as a decline in regenerative capacity. Adult stem cells, responsible for replenishing cells in muscles, skin, and other organs, lose vigor as we age. Their diminished ability to proliferate and differentiate leads to slower healing and tissue maintenance. This decline not only impacts our physical resilience but also influences vulnerability to chronic diseases.

Another critical aspect is the alteration in intercellular communication. Cells constantly signal to each other via chemical messengers, coordinating growth, immune responses, and metabolism. Aging disrupts these communication networks, often promoting pro-inflammatory states and impairing hormonal regulation. These systemic changes contribute to the increased susceptibility to disorders such as insulin resistance, cardiovascular diseases, and impaired immune responses.

While the biological picture of aging may sound daunting, it's important to recognize that aging is not a predetermined fate etched in stone. Instead, it represents a dynamic continuum influenced by genetic factors, environment, and, crucially, behavior. By understanding the underlying mechanisms, you gain a roadmap of where intervention is most effective—whether that's protecting DNA, optimizing mitochondrial function, or clearing damaged cells through targeted strategies.

Science has uncovered that many components of aging are interlinked. For example, improving mitochondrial health not only supports energy production but reduces oxidative stress, helping preserve DNA integrity and protein homeostasis. Similarly, enhancing autophagy not only clears damaged proteins but can also rejuvenate stem cell function. So, a holistic approach that targets multiple aging processes promises the greatest impact on longevity.

Importantly, this section aims not to overwhelm with detail but to inspire a shift in perspective. Aging is a biological process largely shaped by cellular maintenance and damage management. If we can tip the balance toward repair and preservation, functional decline slows, and healthspan extends. This outlook rekindles hope and motivates actionable steps that integrate seamlessly into daily life.

In the chapters ahead, you will explore practical strategies to harness these insights. From nutrition to exercise, sleep optimization to stress management, each intervention taps into these foundational biological principles. By aligning lifestyle choices with biology, it becomes possible to influence how gracefully and vibrantly we age.

Knowledge about the biological roots of aging empowers you to take control, transforming aging from a mysterious inevitability into a manageable, malleable process. When you grasp the cellular orchestration behind it, you don't just pass time—you actively shape your trajectory toward a longer, healthier, and more fulfilling life.

Key Markers of Healthspan

When we talk about longevity, it's easy to focus on lifespan—how long someone lives. But a longer life alone isn't the true goal. What really matters is healthspan, the period during which we stay vibrant, independent, and free from chronic illness. Extending healthspan means adding quality years, not just more years. It's about maintaining strength, sharpness, and resilience as time goes on, so those extra years feel worth living.

Determining and tracking key markers of healthspan gives us vital insight into how well our bodies are aging. These markers act like signposts, indicating how effectively our systems function, how well we resist disease, and how much vitality remains. Unlike arbitrary age, which ticks away at a constant rate, healthspan markers can fluctuate and improve with intentional lifestyle choices. That's empowering. It means the state of your health decades from now isn't set in stone today.

One of the most reliable markers is cardiovascular health. The heart and blood vessels have a tremendous impact on overall well-being, affecting oxygen delivery, endurance, and energy levels. When arteries stiffen or blood pressure rises, the risk for heart disease, stroke, and cognitive decline climbs dramatically. By monitoring factors like resting heart rate, blood pressure, and arterial flexibility, we can gauge cardiovascular vitality, which is a cornerstone of prolonged health. Engaging in consistent physical activity, reducing inflammation through diet, and managing stress play key roles in keeping this system robust.

Muscle mass and strength also stand out as crucial healthspan indicators. It's well-documented that muscle naturally declines with age, and losing just a small percentage annually can make daily activities like climbing stairs or carrying groceries a struggle. More importantly, diminished muscle strength correlates directly with frailty, falls, and loss of independence. Preserving lean muscle through resistance training and adequate protein intake not only extends physical capabilities but promotes metabolic health and glucose regulation. The body's ability to move powerfully and fluidly fundamentally shapes the experience of aging well.

Beyond the muscles and heart lies another critical measure: metabolic function. Insulin sensitivity, glucose regulation, and lipid profiles collectively reflect how efficiently the body uses energy. Poor metabolic health often leads to type 2 diabetes, obesity, and a host of other conditions linked to early mortality. Fortunately, lifestyle interventions such as balanced nutrition, regular exercise, and stress reduction have profound effects on improving metabolic markers. By keeping this system in check, we reduce the wear and tear that accelerates aging inside every cell.

Cognitive health is an equally vital yet often overlooked marker of healthspan. Memory, attention, processing speed, and executive function shape our ability to live independently and meaningfully. Cognitive decline can start subtly decades before symptoms become noticeable, so tracking mental acuity through regular assessments offers a window into brain aging. Activities that stimulate neuroplasticity, emotional well-being, and consistent quality sleep all contribute to preserving this essence of self. The brain's resilience influences not just lifespan but the richness of our lived experience.

Another essential but less tangible marker is inflammation, often described as one of the root causes of aging. Chronic low-grade inflammation silently damages tissue, impairs organ function, and fuels diseases ranging from arthritis to cardiovascular disease and even some cancers. Biomarkers like C-reactive protein (CRP) levels give us a glimpse into our inflammatory state. Lowering inflammation through diet rich in antioxidants, regular movement, and stress-management strategies supports body-wide repair mechanisms, thereby extending healthspan in a subtle yet profound way.

Immune system integrity also forms a significant pillar of sustained health. As we age, immune responses generally weaken—a phenomenon called immunosenescence—making infections harder to fight and vaccinations less effective. Monitoring markers such as white blood cell counts, antibody production, and the balance of immune cell types informs us about the system's robustness. Supporting immunity goes beyond avoiding illness; it ensures ongoing surveillance against abnormal cells and helps keep chronic disease at bay. Lifestyle habits that nurture gut health, adequate sleep, and moderate physical activity broaden this defense network.

Bone density deserves mention as a vital healthspan criterion. Osteoporosis and fractures disproportionately affect older adults, often leading to reduced mobility and autonomy. Strong, healthy bones provide the structural foundation for an active and engaged life. Regular weight-bearing exercises, sufficient calcium and vitamin D intake, and avoiding smoking and excessive alcohol consumption contribute markedly to maintaining bone strength. These measures lessen the likelihood of debilitating injury and preserve the freedom movement brings.

A final major marker to consider involves hormonal balance. Hormones regulate countless processes, including metabolism, mood, muscle growth, and immune function. Throughout aging, declines or imbalances in hormones like growth hormone, testosterone, estrogen, and cortisol can manifest as fatigue, muscle loss, cognitive fog, and increased disease susceptibility. While hormone replacement therapies are sometimes appropriate, lifestyle factors such as stress management, adequate sleep, and balanced nutrition often support more natural stability. Equilibrium in this complex system correlates strongly with sustained vitality and well-being.

It's important to remember that these markers don't exist in isolation. They interconnect to form an intricate web of health, where improvement or decline in one area ripples throughout the body. That's why a holistic approach to monitoring healthspan pays off. Addressing cardiovascular fitness simultaneously boosts metabolic health, muscle strength supports bone density, and reduced inflammation helps preserve cognitive function. Pursuing balanced, well-rounded habits creates positive synergies that multiply benefits.

Measurement and regular check-ins on these markers empower proactive steps. Knowing where you stand allows you to tailor interventions, prioritize areas needing attention, and track progress clearly over time. This isn't about perfection or chasing unattainable immortality. It's about cultivating habits that encourage your body's natural resilience and keeping that internal clock ticking well into advanced years. Each small gain contributes to greater freedom, purpose, and joy in how you age.

Key markers of healthspan offer more than clinical data—they provide motivation and tangible targets. They convert abstract desires for longevity into concrete goals: lowering blood pressure, increasing muscle strength, sharpening memory, reducing inflammation. These goals are achievable, measurable, and tied directly to everyday choices. Leaning into these indicators transforms aging from a passive drifting away into an active journey of empowerment and possibility.

In the next chapters, we'll dive deeper into practical strategies and science-backed interventions that influence these markers. But understanding what to track and why lays the foundation for informed, intentional action. The quest for extended healthspan is a call to live intentionally, respecting the fragile yet remarkably durable nature of the human body. Each step forward can add years of vibrant life, turning time into an ally, not an enemy.

Chapter Three
NUTRITION STRATEGIES FOR EXTENDED LIFE

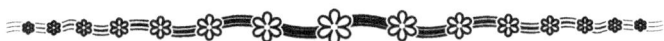

Navigating the path to a longer, healthier life often begins on our plates, where the choices we make daily ripple through our biology in profound ways. Embracing nutrition strategies that reduce chronic inflammation and optimize metabolic health forms the cornerstone of lasting vitality. It's not about restrictive eating but about intelligently selecting foods that not only nourish but also protect the body from the wear and tear of time—those vibrant vegetables, whole grains, and healthy fats that fuel cellular repair and resilience. Integrating mindful eating practices, which honor natural hunger cues and promote metabolic flexibility, encourages a sustainable rhythm that supports longevity without sacrificing the joy of food. By tuning into these nourishing habits, you're not just adding years to your life—you're enhancing the quality of each moment lived, empowering your body to thrive well beyond what many consider its prime.

ANTI-INFLAMMATORY FOODS AND LONGEVITY

Inflammation is a natural response by the body to injury or infection, designed to protect and heal. However, chronic inflammation – the kind that lingers quietly beneath the surface – has been linked to a variety of age-related diseases including heart disease, diabetes, and Alzheimer's. This low-grade, persistent inflammation accelerates the aging process at a cellular level, damaging tissues and organs over time. The good news is that dietary choices can profoundly influence inflammation, either fueling it or taming it. This is why focusing on anti-inflammatory foods isn't just about reducing discomfort in the short term; it's a foundational strategy for extending life and maintaining vitality.

Anti-inflammatory foods work because they contain compounds that directly interact with the body's inflammatory pathways. Phytochemicals, antioxidants, and healthy fats help regulate immune function and reduce oxidative stress, both of which contribute to healing and longevity. When you consistently eat foods rich in these compounds, you're not just avoiding harm—you're actively promoting a cellular environment that supports repair and resilience. This creates a powerful ripple effect, strengthening your defenses against chronic diseases that typically shorten lifespan.

At the heart of an anti-inflammatory diet are whole, minimally processed foods that have stood the test of time. Vegetables like kale, spinach, and broccoli are packed with flavonoids and carotenoids, which play vital roles in calming inflammation and neutralizing free radicals. Berries, bursting with anthocyanins, not only satisfy a sweet craving but also protect blood vessels and brain cells as we age. Incorporating a colorful variety of these plant-based foods ensures a broad spectrum of nutrients working in harmony to preserve health and longevity.

Omega-3 fatty acids deserve special attention in the conversation about anti-inflammatory foods. Found primarily in fatty fish such as salmon, mackerel, and sardines, these essential fats actively reduce the production of pro-inflammatory molecules. They also help maintain the integrity of cell membranes, which is crucial for optimal immune function. Plant sources like walnuts, chia seeds, and flaxseeds provide a precursor to these fats and contribute beneficially, too. Swapping out saturated and trans fats with omega-3 rich options creates an internal environment less prone to chronic inflammation and the diseases that follow.

Herbs and spices offer an often-overlooked but potent anti-inflammatory boost. Turmeric, with its active compound curcumin, has been extensively studied for its capacity to inhibit molecules that drive inflammation. Ginger works in a similar way, soothing the gut and reducing markers of systemic inflammation. These natural remedies complement a healthy diet and can easily be incorporated into meals or teas, making anti-inflammatory eating both effective and flavorful. Not only do they reduce inflammation, but they also provide antioxidants that refresh and protect cells.

Some may think that simply cutting out known inflammatory foods is enough, but proactive inclusion of anti-inflammatory foods makes the biggest difference. It's not just about what you avoid—such as refined sugars, excessive alcohol, and processed meats—but about what you embrace. Prioritizing nutrient-dense choices that feed your cells the right building blocks is a form of self-investment that pays dividends in the form of longer, healthier years. A lifestyle built around anti-inflammatory eating patterns shifts the body from a state of chronic damage to one of repair and longevity.

The Mediterranean diet, often hailed for its health benefits, is a prime example of an anti-inflammatory approach that translates into longer life expectancy. It emphasizes olive oil, nuts, whole grains, fruits, vegetables, and moderate fish consumption—all rich in anti-inflammatory components. This way of eating not only lowers inflammation but also supports cardiovascular health, cognitive function, and metabolic balance. Studies have repeatedly demonstrated that communities embracing this diet tend to enjoy longer lifespans with fewer chronic illnesses.

It's important to recognize that anti-inflammatory foods do more than just suppress harmful pathways—they also enhance the gut microbiome, a crucial player in immune regulation and inflammation control. Fiber-rich foods such as legumes, whole grains, and fruits act as fuel for beneficial gut bacteria. These microbes in turn produce metabolites that reduce intestinal inflammation and promote barrier function.

31

The connection between the gut and longevity is increasingly clear: a healthy microbiome means a balanced immune response, fewer inflammatory triggers, and a firmer foundation for life extension.

Incorporating anti-inflammatory foods doesn't require drastic changes or expensive supplements. Simple swaps like replacing butter with extra virgin olive oil, choosing whole fruits over sugary snacks, or adding a handful of nuts to your salad every day can lead to meaningful reductions in inflammation. What's crucial is consistency and variety, which together maximize the range and potency of anti-inflammatory nutrients your body receives. Over time, these dietary habits accumulate, creating a resilient internal environment buffered from the wear and tear of aging.

Beyond the foods themselves, how you prepare and combine them can influence their anti-inflammatory power. Cooking methods like steaming, roasting, or lightly sautéing preserve nutrients better than deep frying or charring, which can increase oxidative stress. Pairing vitamin C-rich foods with plant-based iron sources improves absorption and supports immune function, indirectly helping to reduce inflammatory stress. Spices like black pepper can even increase the bioavailability of beneficial compounds such as curcumin, amplifying their impact. These small details speak to the broader principle that longevity nutrition is as much an art as a science.

Embracing an anti-inflammatory food philosophy is not just about extending years to your life—it's about adding life to your years. Reduced inflammation is associated with better mobility, clearer cognition, and a decreased risk of debilitating diseases that rob people of their independence. This holistic approach aligns with the deep human need for vitality and meaningful engagement, qualities that money or advanced technology can't replicate. The decision to feed yourself in this way becomes an act of reclaiming your future from the premature effects of aging.

Finally, it's worth noting that adopting an anti-inflammatory diet cultivates mindfulness around eating. When you think about the healing properties of your food and choose ingredients thoughtfully, your relationship with your diet transforms. This mindset shift fosters a greater appreciation for nourishment and encourages other healthy behaviors—a virtuous cycle that supports sustained longevity. Through anti-inflammatory eating, you effectively build a nutritional foundation strong enough to withstand the biological pressures of time, allowing you to thrive, not just survive.

THE ROLE OF CALORIC RESTRICTION AND FASTING

In the search for longer, healthier lives, caloric restriction and fasting have emerged as two of the most intriguing nutritional strategies. These approaches aren't about extreme dieting or fad trends; they tap into deep biological mechanisms that influence aging and disease risk. While the idea of eating less might sound counterintuitive when we're often told to fuel our bodies adequately, the science tells a compelling story about how reducing caloric intake can extend lifespan and improve overall health.

Caloric restriction, in its simplest form, means reducing daily calorie intake without causing malnutrition. It's not about starving yourself but rather eating smart, cutting down excess while still getting the nutrients you need. Research in animals—ranging from worms to primates—has consistently shown that cutting calories by about 20 to 40 percent extends lifespan and delays the onset of age-related diseases. These findings have sparked significant interest in applying similar principles to humans.

One powerful reason caloric restriction works is that it slows down metabolic processes that otherwise lead to cellular damage over time. When calorie intake is reduced, the body undergoes a series of beneficial adaptations. These include improvements in insulin sensitivity, reductions in inflammatory molecules, and enhanced cellular repair mechanisms. This means your body becomes more efficient at handling stress at the cellular level, essentially making the tissues and organs more resilient against the wear and tear of aging.

Fasting, which can be seen as a variant or complement to caloric restriction, involves deliberately abstaining from food for specified periods. Unlike continuous calorie limitation, fasting cycles between periods of eating and not eating, giving the body a break from constant digestion. Intermittent fasting schedules, like the popular 16:8 method (16 hours fasting, 8 hours eating window), or alternate-day fasting, have gained traction for their ability to trigger similar longevity pathways seen in caloric restriction.

The physiological changes fasting induces mirror many of those seen with caloric restriction. Among the most important is the activation of autophagy—a self-cleaning process where cells remove damaged components and recycle them. This cleanup operation is vital for maintaining cellular health and function, reducing the risk of diseases such as cancer, neurodegeneration, and metabolic disorders.

Importantly, both caloric restriction and fasting promote hormonal shifts that favor longevity. For example, insulin and insulin-like growth factor-1 (IGF-1) levels typically decrease, which has been linked to slower aging and reduced cancer risk. At the same time, molecules like adiponectin increase, supporting improved metabolism and anti-inflammatory effects. These hormonal changes set into motion a cascade of molecular events that protect DNA, improve mitochondrial function, and reduce oxidative stress.

While the benefits sound appealing, it's crucial to approach these strategies thoughtfully. Overdoing caloric restriction or fasting without proper nutritional planning can backfire, causing muscle loss, weakened immunity, or nutrient deficiencies. The goal isn't deprivation but balance—reducing excess while maintaining vitality.

For health-conscious individuals, the question becomes how to incorporate these practices sustainably. Fasting schedules like time-restricted eating often offer a manageable entry point. Many find benefits simply by narrowing their daily eating window, without obsessively counting calories or drastically changing what they eat. This flexibility helps create lasting habits rather than temporary fixes.

Moreover, the timing of eating matters. Aligning food intake with circadian rhythms—when the body naturally expects to digest and metabolize food—can amplify the effects of fasting and caloric restriction. Consuming meals earlier in the day, and avoiding late-night snacks, supports better metabolic health and complements these longevity strategies.

Individuals with certain medical conditions or nutritional needs should consult healthcare providers before adopting rigorous fasting or caloric restriction plans. Pregnancy, diabetes, or eating disorders, for example, require specialized approaches to avoid harm. But for most people, these interventions can be adapted safely, personalized according to lifestyle, and combined with nutrient-dense foods to maximize benefit.

It's also encouraging to note that the longevity dividends of caloric restriction and fasting go beyond lifespan extension. Many people report improvements in energy levels, mental clarity, mood stabilization, and better sleep—all factors that enhance quality of life as we age. The science suggests these aren't just side effects but integral parts of the underlying biology that makes us healthier longer.

While we await large-scale, long-term human studies to fully understand the extent of these strategies' impact, the existing evidence and evolutionary logic provide solid footing. Human bodies evolved through periods of feast and famine, and modern constant food availability is a new phenomenon that our biology continues to adapt to. Embracing periods of reduced intake, whether through controlled calories or fasting, reconnects us with these ancient rhythms.

Importantly, caloric restriction and fasting are not about punishment or rigid rules; they're tools for reclaiming control over aging processes that often feel inevitable. Adopting these practices can be empowering—helping you tune into your body's signals, improve metabolic health, and extend your healthspan so you spend more years enjoying life fully.

Incorporating caloric restriction and fasting doesn't mean you need to live on salads or skip celebrations. Instead, think of it as creating purposeful pauses and moderation. It's about quality as much as quantity—choosing nutrient-rich foods, avoiding constant grazing, and respecting your body's natural cycles. These shifts, though subtle at first, can ripple out to profound, long-lasting changes in how you age.

To get started, consider small, manageable adjustments rather than radical overhaul. Try shortening your eating window by an hour or two, experimenting with one or two fasting days per week, or modestly reducing portion sizes. Pay attention to how your body responds, how your energy fluctuates, and use that feedback to tailor your approach.

The role of caloric restriction and fasting in longevity isn't a secret or a mysterious formula; it's an invitation to explore what our bodies are truly capable of when given time and rest to heal and adapt. When combined with other nutrition strategies and a balanced lifestyle, these practices can be the foundation for a vibrant, extended life.

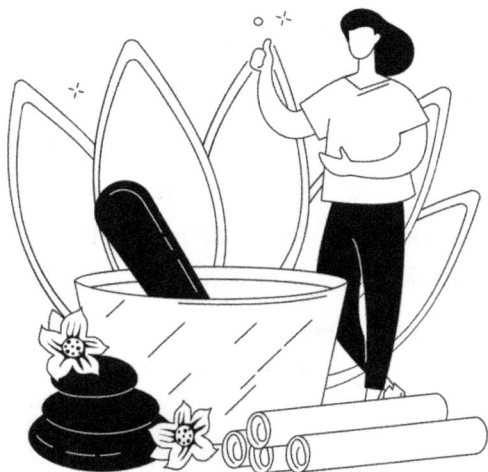

Chapter Four
EXERCISE AND PHYSICAL VITALITY

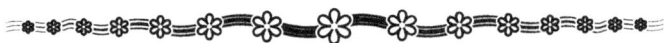

Movement is far more than a daily task; it's a cornerstone for a longer, more vibrant life that fuels both body and mind. Engaging regularly in physical activity isn't about punishing your body with endless hours at the gym—it's a deliberate, potent strategy to bolster muscle strength, improve cardiovascular function, and ignite resilience against the wear of aging. Exercise sharpens metabolic health, enhances mitochondrial efficiency, and even sparks beneficial cellular adaptations that promote longevity. When you prioritize consistent, well-rounded exercise, you're laying down a foundation that supports energy, agility, and wellness throughout every stage of life. This vitality doesn't just add years to your lifespan; it adds life to your years, empowering you to move confidently and fully, meeting the future with strength and vitality.

STRENGTH TRAINING FOR LIFELONG HEALTH

Strength training stands as one of the most powerful tools you can use to extend both your lifespan and healthspan. It's often mistaken as something relevant only for athletes or young adults, but the truth is, building and maintaining muscle is a critical factor for vitality at any age. Muscle strength affects everything from metabolic health and mobility to mental resilience and even longevity itself. In fact, those who engage in regular strength training show improved survival rates compared to those who don't, partly because muscle mass plays a key role in protecting us against age-related diseases.

The biology behind why strength training matters so much begins with how muscle tissue influences insulin sensitivity, inflammation, and hormonal balance. When you work your muscles against resistance, you're not just making them bulkier; you're actually fostering cellular mechanisms that slow down the aging process. Muscle cells produce beneficial substances known as myokines, which have anti-inflammatory properties and communicate with other organs, including the brain and liver. This communication network helps regulate metabolism, prevent chronic diseases, and sustain energy levels throughout the day.

Another critical element is the preservation of bone density. Without regular strength training, bones lose their density as we age, increasing the risk of fractures and osteoporosis. The mechanical stress applied during resistance exercises triggers bone remodeling and growth, much like muscle adaptation. This effect is especially valuable because fractures can severely impact independence and quality of life in older adults. Strength training becomes, therefore, not just an anti-aging strategy but a crucial protective measure for lifelong mobility.

One of the most compelling reasons to invest in strength training lies in its impact on functional capacity. Everyday activities such as climbing stairs, carrying groceries, or even getting up from a chair all depend on muscular strength and coordination. Age-related muscle loss, known as sarcopenia, is a major contributor to frailty and falls, which are among the leading causes of injury in older populations. Regularly challenging your muscles with strength exercises reverses muscle decline and improves balance and coordination, reducing the risk of injuries that can drastically shorten healthy years.

What's remarkable about strength training is how adaptable it is—there's no one-size-fits-all approach. Whether you prefer free weights, resistance bands, bodyweight exercises, or machines, you can tailor a routine that suits your preferences and physical condition. Starting even with moderate resistance loads can stimulate muscle growth and strength improvements; you don't need to lift heavy weights or train for hours. Consistency and progressive overload—gradually increasing demands on your muscles—are what drive results. This adaptability is crucial, as sustainability remains a key factor in lifelong exercise adherence.

The mental and neurological benefits of strength training also deserve attention. Emerging research highlights resistance exercise as a potent stimulator of brain health, promoting the release of growth factors that aid in brain plasticity and cognitive function. This isn't just about memory or focus; maintaining mental sharpness supports decision-making skills essential for managing health behaviors, medication adherence, and social engagement. Strength training, therefore, feeds into the larger ecosystem of a resilient mind-body connection, essential for prolonged wellbeing.

Integrating strength training into your life also brings metabolic perks. Muscle tissue is metabolically active, meaning it burns calories even at rest. As you gain muscle, you increase your basal metabolic rate, which helps regulate body weight and reduces the risk of metabolic syndrome, diabetes, and cardiovascular disease. The hormonal environment created by regular resistance exercise contributes to better appetite regulation and improved lipid profiles. These effects compound over time, reinforcing a positive feedback loop where strength supports health, and health supports strength.

Despite all these benefits, strength training is surprisingly underutilized, especially by those over 50. Part of the hesitation comes from misconceptions about safety or complexity. The reality is that, with appropriate guidance and progression, strength training can be one of the safest forms of exercise—better yet, it's one of the most empowering. You're actively reclaiming control over your physical capabilities and defying the expectations often associated with aging.

That sense of agency can inspire greater confidence to take on challenges beyond the gym.

You don't need a gym membership or fancy equipment to start. Even simple bodyweight exercises like squats, push-ups, and lunges provide significant strength benefits. Using resistance bands or household items like water bottles as weights can make these workouts more challenging without requiring special tools. The key is to prioritize form and gradually increase intensity over weeks and months. Short, focused sessions done two to three times a week can yield meaningful improvements in muscle strength and quality of life.

It's also important to view strength training as part of a broader lifestyle strategy rather than an isolated task. Nutrition, rest, and recovery all intersect with your ability to build and maintain muscle. Adequate protein intake is crucial to support muscle repair, but equally vital are periods of rest that allow muscles to rebuild stronger. Overtraining can backfire, leading to injury or burnout. Finding that balance comes with paying attention to your body's signals—soreness, fatigue, and energy levels—and adjusting your approach accordingly.

Safety and proper technique are paramount, especially if you're new to strength training or returning after a long break. Consider working with a qualified trainer at first to develop a routine that matches your personal goals and limitations. They can help you learn movement patterns that protect your joints and reduce injury risk. Over time, the confidence gained from mastering these exercises can empower you to take more ownership of your fitness journey.

Strength training also provides community and social engagement opportunities that can bolster mental health and adherence. Group classes or small workout groups create connections and accountability, which are proven motivators for maintaining exercise routines. These social connections contribute to emotional wellbeing and resilience, both of which are linked to longer, healthier lives. So, while the physical benefits of strength training are essential, the psychological and social rewards should not be overlooked.

Ultimately, strength training for lifelong health is about more than muscle—it's about creating a foundation for vibrant aging. It's about keeping your body capable, your mind sharp, and your spirit confident in its ability to meet life's demands. By embracing regular resistance exercise, you're signaling a commitment to yourself, an investment in years of quality living that far outweighs the time spent lifting weights.

The narrative around aging is shifting. Strength training disrupts the expectation that decline is inevitable and irreversible. Instead, it offers a blueprint for sustainable vitality that supports you—not just in adding years to life but life to your years. It's a practice that echoes deeply with the core aim of longevity: thriving with purpose, passion, and power.

CARDIOVASCULAR FITNESS AND LONGEVITY BENEFITS

Stepping beyond the basics of exercise, cardiovascular fitness stands out as a cornerstone for extending both lifespan and healthspan. It's not just about having a strong heart or lungs—it's about the profound effects that regular cardiovascular activity has on nearly every system in the body. When we talk about longevity strategies, the role of cardiovascular fitness is paramount. It's the engine that powers your body's resilience against age-related decline, chronic illnesses, and cognitive deterioration.

At its core, cardiovascular fitness refers to how efficiently your heart, lungs, and blood vessels work together to supply oxygen to your tissues during sustained physical activity. Activities like brisk walking, jogging, cycling, and swimming all boost this fitness, training your heart to pump more blood with fewer beats, improving oxygen delivery and utilization. Over time, this efficiency cascades into reduced wear on the cardiovascular system, lowering your risk of hypertension, coronary artery disease, stroke, and a spectrum of other diseases that frequently shorten lifespan.

But this goes far beyond simply strengthening the heart muscle. One of the remarkable benefits of cardiovascular fitness is its effect on the vascular system itself. Regular aerobic exercise promotes the formation of collateral blood vessels, improving circulation and reducing the chance of blockages. Additionally, it increases the flexibility of arteries, which tends to decline with age, making your blood vessels more durable and less susceptible to damage. This vascular health is directly linked to lower risks of heart attacks and strokes, two leading causes of mortality worldwide.

More interestingly, cardiovascular exercise fosters a powerful anti-inflammatory environment within the body. Chronic inflammation is a known accelerator of the aging process, contributing to the progression of multiple diseases such as diabetes, Alzheimer's, and certain cancers. By engaging in regular aerobic activity, you help modulate immune responses, calming systemic inflammation and supporting healthier aging. This is one of the reasons why populations with high levels of physical activity tend to enjoy longer, healthier lives.

Looking deeper into the mechanisms, cardiovascular fitness enhances mitochondrial function and biogenesis. Mitochondria are often called the "powerhouses" of the cell because they generate the energy cells need to operate. Aging is closely linked to mitochondrial decline, which impairs energy metabolism and increases cellular stress. By challenging your cardiovascular system through consistent aerobic exercise, you stimulate mitochondrial growth and efficiency, effectively rebooting your cellular engines. The result? Greater vitality and increased resistance to age-related fatigue and degenerative conditions.

Another vital aspect is the impact on metabolic health. Cardiovascular fitness improves insulin sensitivity, meaning your body uses glucose more effectively, preventing damage caused by elevated blood sugar levels. Given that metabolic disorders like type 2 diabetes drastically shorten healthspan, optimizing cardiovascular function plays a critical preventative role. As blood sugar regulation improves, so does lipid metabolism, helping maintain a healthier balance between "good" and "bad" cholesterol.

Beyond the physiological, cardiovascular fitness carries significant psychological benefits that ripple out into longevity. You've likely heard about the "runner's high," but the mood-enhancing effects go much deeper. Regular aerobic exercise increases the release of endorphins and brain-derived neurotrophic factor (BDNF). BDNF is particularly important because it supports neuroplasticity, or the brain's ability to adapt and grow new connections, which is crucial for cognitive resilience as we age. Mental sharpness and emotional well-being feed into longevity by encouraging an active, social, and engaged lifestyle.

When exploring the landscape of longevity interventions, it stands out that cardiovascular fitness operates as a multifaceted safeguard—reducing risks, boosting energy, and supporting mental health in tandem. The best part? It's accessible. You don't need a gym membership or specialized equipment. Walking briskly around your neighborhood or engaging in any consistent aerobic activity can trigger these extensive benefits.

There's also compelling evidence from epidemiological studies linking higher levels of cardiovascular fitness with significantly reduced mortality risk. For example, those maintaining good aerobic capacity have been shown to live, on average, 5 to 7 years longer than sedentary individuals. The protective effects are dose-dependent, meaning the more you invest in cardiovascular health, the more you stand to gain. And even moderate increases in fitness, especially for those previously inactive, lead to remarkable improvements.

It's important to recognize, though, that the goal isn't to become a marathon runner overnight. Longevity stems from consistent, sustained effort over time. Integrating cardiovascular exercise into your weekly routine in ways that feel sustainable—whether through dancing, gardening, or cycling—will pay dividends not just in years added to lifespan, but years added to quality of life.

Moreover, cardiovascular fitness creates a foundation that amplifies the benefits of other longevity practices. A well-tuned cardiovascular system enhances recovery from strength training, supports better sleep, and energizes the mental focus required for stress management and dietary discipline. The synergistic effect means you're not just adding one healthy habit; you're unlocking a lifestyle optimized for endurance, vitality, and joy.

In adopting a mindset that embraces cardiovascular fitness as a pillar of longevity, consider setting achievable goals that blend challenge and enjoyment. Track your progress through simple metrics—how far you walk, how you feel during and after activity, or your resting heart rate. These indicators provide immediate feedback and motivate you to keep advancing. Remember, the journey of longevity is a marathon in which each step, each beat of your heart, counts toward a future of sustained health.

In sum, cardiovascular fitness is a non-negotiable element in the pursuit of a long and vibrant life. It fosters not just the systemic health that protects against chronic diseases, but also the cellular and cognitive resilience needed to thrive into advanced age. Cultivating it doesn't require drastic change, only a commitment to move your body regularly in ways that raise your heart rate and connect breath with motion. When you consistently honor this relationship with your cardiovascular system, you are laying down one of the strongest foundations for enduring wellness and longevity.

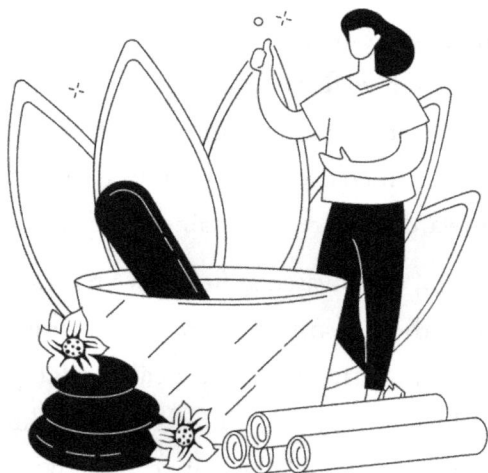

Chapter Five
MENTAL HEALTH AND COGNITIVE LONGEVITY

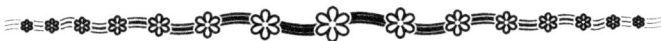

Maintaining a sharp, resilient mind is just as critical as caring for the body when it comes to living longer and better. The brain thrives on challenge, connection, and calm; neglecting these can accelerate decline, but nurturing them can unlock remarkable cognitive vitality well into later years. It's not enough to simply avoid stress—learning to manage it effectively rewires our response to adversity and buffers us against mental wear and tear. Embracing activities that actively engage the brain sparks neuroplasticity, the brain's incredible ability to adapt, which keeps memory and problem-solving skills vibrant over time. By prioritizing mental wellness as a cornerstone of longevity, we build a robust foundation that supports not just a longer life, but one filled with clarity, purpose, and joy.

STRESS MANAGEMENT TECHNIQUES

Stress, often dismissed as a mere nuisance, silently chips away at both mental health and cognitive longevity. Prolonged exposure to stress hormones like cortisol can speed up cognitive aging and impair memory, focus, and emotional regulation. The good news? While you can't eliminate stress completely, you can learn to manage it effectively. Stress management techniques are essential tools in preserving your cognitive vitality and enhancing overall mental well-being.

Consider stress not just as a state of mind but as a complex biological response. When you're overwhelmed, your body enters a fight-or-flight mode, flooding your system with hormones that, over time, wear down the brain's resilience. Managing stress effectively helps maintain the structures of the brain involved in learning and memory, such as the hippocampus, and reduces inflammation—both crucial for longevity. Establishing a daily routine that includes proven stress management practices equips you to face challenges without sacrificing your cognitive health.

One of the most accessible and powerful stress management techniques is focused breathing. Deep, intentional breaths signal your nervous system to shift from the reactive fight-or-flight state to a calmer rest-and-digest mode. You don't have to spend hours meditating; even brief moments of mindful breathing scattered throughout your day can reset your nervous system and curb the cascade of stress hormones. This simple practice grows your tolerance to stress and enhances clarity and emotional balance.

Another approach gaining scientific backing is mindfulness meditation. Beyond the buzzwords, mindfulness trains your brain to remain present, to observe thoughts and feelings without judgment, and to disengage from the cycle of rumination that prolongs stress. Regular mindfulness meditation has been associated with increased gray matter density in brain regions tied to emotional regulation and executive function. This promotes cognitive longevity by fostering mental flexibility and improving your ability to adapt to new challenges.

Physical activity also plays a vital role in stress management. Exercise stimulates the production of endorphins—the body's natural mood elevators—and reduces circulating cortisol levels. Whether it's a brisk walk, yoga, or resistance training, movement provides a practical outlet for anxiety and tension. Engaging multiple times a week with enjoyable physical activities bolsters not only physical vitality but also mental resilience, creating a buffer against the harmful effects of stress.

Sleep, often underappreciated in conversations about stress, is yet another cornerstone. High stress levels disrupt sleep architecture, impairing the restorative cycles necessary for brain repair and memory consolidation. On the flip side, prioritizing quality sleep supports emotional regulation, making stressors feel less overwhelming. Developing a consistent sleep routine, creating a calming pre-bedtime ritual, and limiting electronic distractions can dramatically reduce stress-related cognitive decline.

Beyond individual practices, social connection is a surprisingly potent antidote to stress. Humans are wired for connection, and nurturing meaningful relationships provides emotional support that helps dampen stress responses. Engaging in community activities or simply sharing your thoughts with trusted friends or family members buffers the brain against isolation-induced cognitive decline. Longevity researchers increasingly highlight social engagement as an invisible, but powerful, shield against stress-related memory loss and anxiety.

Techniques that involve creative expression can also ease the burden of stress. Activities such as journaling, painting, or playing music allow an outlet for emotions and offer a shift in perspective. Writing about stressful events, for instance, has been shown to help process emotions and reduce psychological distress. These outlets foster cognitive clarity and emotional balance, further fortifying mental health over the long term.

It's important to recognize that no single technique suits everyone. The key lies in developing a personalized toolkit. Start by experimenting with multiple methods and noting their effects on your mood and mental sharpness. Combining physical, emotional, and cognitive approaches—like pairing regular exercise with mindfulness and social engagement—aids in building a robust defense against the cumulative wear of stress.

Modern life throws countless stressors at us daily, from work pressures to health concerns and unexpected challenges. Neglecting stress management isn't just uncomfortable; it chips away at your brain's ability to function at peak levels, increasing the risk of cognitive decline. However, adopting stress management techniques transcends mere symptom relief. It's about cultivating resilience, fostering a mindset that embraces challenges without being overwhelmed by them.

Science underscores that managing stress doesn't just improve how you feel in the moment; it can literally slow down aspects of brain aging. By keeping chronic inflammation and hormonal imbalances in check, these techniques preserve the integrity of neural pathways and promote neuroplasticity, the brain's ability to rewire itself—a key to maintaining mental sharpness well into old age.

In the grand scheme of longevity, stress management is not an optional luxury but an indispensable pillar. It bridges the gap between living longer and living better. The cognitive gains you achieve aren't abstract concepts but translate into sharper decision-making, richer relationships, and a more vibrant engagement with life. Implementing these techniques means you invest in a future where your mind remains as vital as your body.

Ultimately, stress management is a lifelong commitment and an act of self-compassion. The journey involves ongoing learning, adaptation, and patience. But the payoff—sustained cognitive function, emotional stability, and a sense of control over your mental health—is invaluable. As you incorporate these techniques into your routine, you build a foundation that supports not just longevity, but a meaningful, enriched life.

BRAIN-BOOSTING ACTIVITIES AND NEUROPLASTICITY

As we seek to extend not only our lifespan but also our cognitive vitality, understanding the malleability of the brain becomes essential. Neuroplasticity, the brain's remarkable ability to reorganize itself by forming new neural connections, serves as the foundation for countless brain-boosting activities. Far from being a fixed organ, the brain is dynamic and adaptable, even as we age. This capacity to change keeps cognitive functions sharp and opens doors to lifelong learning and mental resilience.

Engaging in mentally stimulating activities is not just about avoiding cognitive decline—it's about thriving and expanding your mental potential. When you immerse yourself in challenging tasks, whether it's learning a new language, playing a musical instrument, or tackling complex puzzles, you actively promote neural growth. These activities encourage the brain to develop new pathways, enhance synaptic efficiency, and improve communication between different regions. The end result is a more flexible, agile mind equipped to handle everyday demands and unexpected challenges with poise.

It's tempting to think that brain-boosting requires hours of intense focus or specialized knowledge. In reality, simple practices, when performed consistently, wield profound benefits. Reading deeply, engaging in thoughtful conversations, or even exploring unfamiliar cultures and ideas stimulate cognitive networks. The key is novelty and complexity, challenging your brain enough to push beyond comfort zones without overwhelming it.

Recent research underscores that physical and mental exercises work synergistically, but when focusing on mental fitness specifically, variety plays a pivotal role. Exposing yourself to different types of cognitive tasks enhances your brain's adaptability. One day might involve strategic games like chess that demand foresight and planning. Another could be creative writing or drawing, which encourage divergent thinking and imagination. This diversity triggers multiple regions of the brain to activate and continuously adapt, reinforcing neuroplasticity.

Mindfulness practices and meditation also contribute to brain health by fine-tuning attention and emotional regulation. Studies demonstrate that regular meditation can increase gray matter density in areas responsible for memory, learning, and emotional control. These changes correlate with improved focus and a steadier mind, which are crucial for mental longevity in a world brimming with distractions and stress.

What's equally encouraging is that neuroplasticity does not dwindle completely with age—it simply requires more deliberate effort to engage. Aging brains may not be as fast to form new pathways, but they certainly retain the potential to rewire and reorganize. The implication is clear: it's never too late to start prioritizing brain-boosting activities. In fact, adopting such habits later in life still improves cognitive reserve, delaying the onset and severity of conditions like dementia.

Technology can be a powerful ally in this journey. Interactive brain-training apps and digitally enhanced learning platforms provide structured yet adaptable challenges tailored to individual cognitive profiles.

They offer measurable progress and encourage sustained engagement. However, it's important to approach them as supplements rather than replacements for rich, real-world experiences and social interactions.

Social connection itself stands as one of the most potent cognitive enhancers. Conversations, group problem-solving, and shared learning experiences create complex neural engagement that solitary activities may lack. The dynamic back-and-forth of human interaction fosters emotion-driven learning that cements memory better than rote repetition. These exchanges spark release of neurochemicals like dopamine and oxytocin, which not only reinforce learning but also promote mental well-being.

Nutrition plays a subtle but important role in supporting neuroplasticity. Nutrients such as omega-3 fatty acids, antioxidants, and vitamins enhance synaptic function and protect against cognitive decline by reducing oxidative stress and inflammation in brain tissues. While specific dietary strategies are detailed elsewhere, it's worth noting that brain-boosting activities flourish best when paired with a diet that nourishes sharpness and longevity at the cellular level.

Adopting a lifestyle that prioritizes brain health demands more than isolated acts; it requires an integrated approach where mental activity, physical movement, social engagement, and nutrition intersect. Neuroplasticity thrives in this ecosystem. Picture your brain as a garden: the activities you choose are seeds, the lifestyle your sunlight and water. The more diversely and consistently you tend to it, the richer your cognitive landscape will become.

Some might wonder if brain training is simply a trend without lasting benefits. Yet decades of studies prove otherwise. The brain's plastic nature reveals that sustained mental engagement builds cognitive reserve, boosting memory, problem-solving, and processing speed. This reserve acts as a buffer against age-related changes, allowing individuals to maintain independence and quality of life longer than previously assumed possible.

Translating this knowledge into action means shifting from passive consumption—like endlessly scrolling through social media or binge-watching television—to actively challenging the mind. Investing time in puzzles, strategy games, learning new skills, or even volunteering for mentally demanding tasks can be transformative. The effort pays dividends in clear thinking, emotional balance, and resilience against cognitive decline.

Creating your personalized brain-boosting routine can start with small, enjoyable steps. Choose activities that intrigue you rather than forcing a regimen that feels like a chore. Consistency matters far more than intensity. Over weeks and months, confidence will build alongside cognitive improvements, fostering enthusiasm for deeper engagement.

Keep in mind that rest and recovery are part of this equation too. The brain consolidates learning during downtime, so adequate sleep and moments of mental rest reinforce the gains from active periods. Balancing stimulation with relaxation optimizes neuroplastic processes, allowing new connections to strengthen and become permanent.

Ultimately, embracing brain-boosting activities is about reclaiming agency over aging. It's a commitment to lifelong growth, curiosity, and the belief in your brain's ability to evolve. The joy of mastering new skills, the satisfaction of solving a difficult problem, and the meaningful connections forged along the way are part of a vibrant, extended mental lifespan. These endeavors not only fill your years with vitality but help ensure that your inner world stays as rich and dynamic as the life you've worked to build.

Chapter Six
SLEEP'S IMPACT ON LIFESPAN

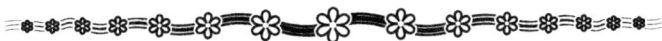

≈·❀·❀·❀═❀═❀═❀═❀═❀═❀═❀═❀═❀·❀·❀·❀·❀·❀·≈

Sleep isn't just a passive state of rest—it's a dynamic, essential process that directly shapes how long and how well we live. Quality sleep acts as the body's powerful repair system, clearing out toxins, supporting immune function, and regulating metabolism, all of which play a pivotal role in reducing the risk of chronic disease and premature aging. When we skimp on sleep, we disrupt those vital processes, accelerating wear and tear on our cells and increasing inflammation that can shorten lifespan. But beyond the physical, restorative sleep also nurtures mental resilience, helping maintain cognitive sharpness and emotional balance that sustain a vibrant, engaged life well into our later years. By prioritizing consistent, deep sleep within an optimized environment, we activate a foundation for longevity that compounds daily—making sleep one of the most accessible and effective tools we have to extend both lifespan and vitality.

SLEEP CYCLES AND RECOVERY PROCESSES

When we think about sleep, it's easy to imagine it as just a passive state where the body and mind rest. But in reality, sleep is a dynamic process, cycling through different phases that each play a critical role in physical and mental recovery. Understanding these cycles isn't just a curiosity—it's key to unlocking how sleep influences lifespan and overall health. The way we cycle through these phases every night directly impacts how well our bodies repair, regenerate, and maintain optimal function, ultimately affecting how long and how well we live.

Sleep can be broadly divided into two main types: non-rapid eye movement (NREM) sleep and rapid eye movement (REM) sleep. NREM sleep itself is further broken down into stages ranging from light sleep to deep, slow-wave sleep (SWS). Each night, our body cycles through these stages multiple times, about every 90 to 120 minutes, starting with light sleep before descending into deep sleep and finally moving into REM sleep, where vivid dreaming typically occurs. This cycling is far more than just a biological rhythm— it's a finely tuned mechanism that supports different aspects of recovery and restoration.

Deep sleep, or slow-wave sleep, deserves special attention for anyone interested in longevity. It is during this phase that the body's most potent restorative processes take place. Growth hormone, a key player in tissue repair, muscle growth, and metabolic balance, is released primarily during deep sleep. This hormone not only supports healing from daily wear and tear but also has far-reaching effects on the aging process. Studies suggest that quality and quantity of deep sleep decline as we age, which corresponds with a decrease in growth hormone secretion. This gradual loss can impair the body's ability to recover from damage and maintain youthful function, highlighting why preserving deep sleep is crucial for lifespan extension.

REM sleep has an equally vital role, especially for cognitive health and emotional well-being. During REM, the brain processes memories, consolidates learning, and manages emotional regulation. Though it represents a smaller portion of the overall sleep time,

REM sleep's influence extends to hormone regulation too, including the balance of stress hormones like cortisol. Proper REM sleep can reduce inflammation and help maintain a healthy neuroendocrine system, which otherwise might accelerate aging and increase vulnerability to chronic diseases. Without sufficient REM stages, the brain's ability to recover from daily stress diminishes, potentially shortening functional lifespan and quality of life.

The fascinating part about these cycles is their interdependence. It's not just about spending enough time asleep, but about maintaining a natural rhythm that effectively transitions between NREM and REM stages throughout the night. This rhythmic cycling supports a flow of reparative and regulatory processes, each complementing the other in a continuous loop of restoration. Disruptions in this rhythm—whether from poor sleep habits, irregular schedules, or external disturbances—can throw off this balance, reducing the restorative benefits and contributing to accelerated aging.

Sleep's recovery benefits are intricately linked to cellular repair as well. Research has shown that during certain sleep stages, especially deep sleep, cells ramp up their repair mechanisms—fixing DNA damage, clearing metabolic waste, and reducing oxidative stress. This is critical because accumulated DNA damage and oxidative stress are at the heart of aging and age-related diseases. Effective repair during sleep means fewer errors building up in cells, which translates into a lower risk of chronic conditions like cancer, cardiovascular disease, and neurodegeneration. It's no exaggeration to say that the body's ability to stay youthful hinges largely on the quality of these nightly recovery cycles.

Another key player in this story is the glymphatic system—a waste clearance network in the brain that's particularly active during sleep. This system floods the brain with cerebrospinal fluid during deep sleep, flushing out toxins, including proteins linked to Alzheimer's disease such as beta-amyloid. When sleep cycles are incomplete or disrupted, the glymphatic system can't work efficiently, allowing harmful byproducts to accumulate. This accumulation accelerates brain aging and increases the likelihood of cognitive decline, making the integrity of sleep cycles a frontline defense in maintaining brain health over time.

All of these processes form a blueprint that shows why chronic sleep deprivation or fragmented sleep can have such devastating effects on lifespan. When sleep's usual cyclicality is compromised, the outcomes bleed into every system of the body—immune response weakens, metabolic health deteriorates, inflammation spikes, and the brain loses its capacity to recover fully. Over time, these cascading effects contribute to systemic decline, making sleep disruption a significant risk factor for reduced longevity.

But here's the optimistic part: sleep cycles and recovery processes can be optimized. Just as nutrition and exercise require evidence-based strategies, the same applies to sleep. Supporting a stable and consistent sleep pattern helps reinforce natural cycling through the sleep stages, maximizing restorative benefits. Going beyond just total sleep time, prioritizing uninterrupted progression through NREM and REM stages enhances the body's ability to heal itself, maintain hormone balance, and preserve cognitive function.

Practical steps toward optimizing sleep cycles focus on aligning sleep patterns with natural circadian rhythms. Staying consistent with bedtimes, minimizing exposure to blue light before sleep, and creating a sleep-conducive environment all promote a smooth flow through the stages of sleep. When your body learns to predict and prepare for sleep, it strengthens the physiological processes that encourage deep, restorative phases and sufficient REM periods. Over time, these intentional habits can shift sleep quality to a level where it meaningfully supports longevity.

We also shouldn't overlook the importance of minimizing sleep interruptions. Frequent awakenings break the sleep cycle, fragmenting the night's restorative processes. Quality sleep means not only the correct amount but also sustained periods within each cycle phase. This is why factors like stress, noise, sleep apnea, and substance use impact longevity—they disrupt the uninterrupted flow of recovery during the night. Addressing these issues can transform an ordinary night's sleep into a powerful act of rejuvenation.

Beyond preventing deterioration, healthy sleep cycles actively promote better aging. Individuals who maintain robust sleep patterns show improved markers of healthspan: better immune surveillance, efficient metabolic function, and lower levels of chronic inflammation, all of which contribute to a longer, higher quality life. It's an investment that pays dividends across every organ system, underscoring the need to treat sleep as a foundational pillar of longevity, not just a passive state to be endured.

The journey toward extending lifespan through sleep doesn't necessitate complex interventions or expensive gadgets. Instead, it calls for a deeper appreciation of how the body's natural rhythms govern recovery. By cultivating habits that encourage full, rich sleep cycles, you give your body the best chance to repair, regenerate, and resist the wear and tear of time. This knowledge empowers you to see sleep not as a luxury but as an essential driver of health and longevity.

OPTIMIZING SLEEP ENVIRONMENT FOR LONGEVITY

Good sleep isn't just about clocking enough hours; it's about creating an environment that allows your body and mind to fully recharge. For those focused on extending lifespan and improving quality of life, the connection between a well-crafted sleep environment and longevity can't be overstated. The quality of your sleep environment influences how deeply you rest, how well your body heals, and how effectively your brain clears out toxins accumulated during the day. Improving these factors means you're not just surviving but thriving over the long term.

What makes a sleep environment truly optimal? It starts with understanding that our bodies respond to very specific cues within our surroundings. Temperature, lighting, noise levels, and even the materials you sleep on all feed into how restorative your rest will be. When these elements align with the natural rhythms of your body, your sleep cycles—those all-important patterns of light sleep, deep sleep, and REM—are free to unfold smoothly. Disturbing this balance can derail your nightly recovery and shorten your functional lifespan in subtle but significant ways.

Let's begin with temperature. Humans evolved sleeping in environments cooler than modern heated homes typically provide. Scientific studies suggest that keeping your bedroom temperature around 60 to 67 degrees Fahrenheit supports the body's natural drop in core temperature, which is crucial for initiating sleep and maintaining deep sleep stages. Overheating—even by a few degrees—can fragment your sleep or reduce time spent in slow-wave sleep, the phase when cellular repair and immune system fortification are at their peak.

Next, there's lighting, arguably one of the most powerful controllable factors in sleep quality. Exposure to dim or no light during sleep supports melatonin release, the hormone that signals your body to rest and repair. Bright and blue light emitted from screens or overhead bulbs confuses this system, delaying sleep onset and reducing total restorative sleep. To optimize your environment, switch off electronics at least an hour before bed, or use warm, low-intensity lighting. Blackout curtains or sleep masks add another layer of protection against disruptive streetlights or early morning sun, extending the natural darkness your body craves.

Noise is another subtle saboteur of longevity-focused rest. Unlike the sharp disturbance of a loud alarm or sudden sound, persistent background noise can cause micro-awakenings you might not even remember but that erode sleep quality. White noise machines or fans can help mask erratic sounds and create a consistent soundscape conducive to deep sleep. Some people find natural sounds like rain or ocean waves especially soothing, tapping into evolutionary cues that signal safety and calm.

The surface you sleep on also plays an essential role. Mattresses and pillows that support proper spinal alignment prevent discomfort and avoid tossing throughout the night. Pain and restlessness, even at low levels, interfere with the uninterrupted sleep your body needs for detoxification and repair. Investing in materials that suit your body shape and firmness preference means fewer disturbances and deeper cycles of rejuvenation. Additionally, natural and breathable fabrics for bedding encourage temperature regulation, enhancing overall comfort.

Beyond physical components, the organization and atmosphere of your sleep space contribute to mental relaxation—a cornerstone of sound sleep. A cluttered or chaotic bedroom sends subtle mental signals that can increase stress or alertness, keeping your mind from fully disengaging. Transforming your bedroom into a calm sanctuary, free of work materials and distractions, reinforces an automatic association with rest and recovery. This mental cue primes your nervous system to downshift into parasympathetic dominance, encouraging smoother transitions through the sleep phases that repair and restore vitality.

Given the deep impact of circadian health on longevity, aligning your sleep environment with natural light-dark cycles is priceless. Exposure to bright light during the day, not just outside of the bedroom, programs your internal clock to feel tired when darkness falls. At night, avoiding artificial light allows your body to reach peak melatonin secretion. Over time, this synchronization supports everything from cellular metabolic processes to hormone regulation, all key players in extending healthspan.

Humidity is an often-overlooked aspect of sleep environments. Too dry or too humid air can influence breathing quality, nasal comfort, and skin hydration. Poor air quality or dryness risks interrupting sleep with irritation or congestion. Using humidifiers or air purifiers to maintain an ideal indoor climate can help your respiratory system function effortlessly during sleep, promoting uninterrupted rest and reducing inflammatory responses. Clean air, in particular, helps safeguard lung health and supports the immune system—a powerful ally in longevity.

Sound, light, temperature, and air quality all come together to form the ecosystem of your bedroom. When these elements are optimized, the body can enter and maintain the critical slow-wave and REM sleep phases that support processes like memory consolidation, tissue repair, immune function, and toxin clearance. This isn't just about feeling refreshed the next day; it's about fortifying the biological foundation necessary to stave off age-related diseases and functional decline.

Sleep environment should be seen not as an afterthought, but as a proactive, daily ritual that complements nutrition, exercise, and stress management in the quest for a longer, healthier life.

Even small adjustments—like investing in blackout curtains, setting strict 'screen-off' rules, or upgrading the mattress—can produce outsized benefits over time. When you prioritize these changes, you're sending a clear message to your body and brain: rest is sacred, and you intend to thrive both today and decades from now.

Creating an ideal sleep environment requires mindful awareness and often experimentation. What feels comfortable and relaxing can vary, but the underlying principle remains consistent: your sleep space needs to support uninterrupted cycles of natural rest that nurture repair and resilience. Think of your bedroom as the sanctuary where the body's longevity blueprint is activated every single night—don't make it a place for anything less than profound healing and transformation.

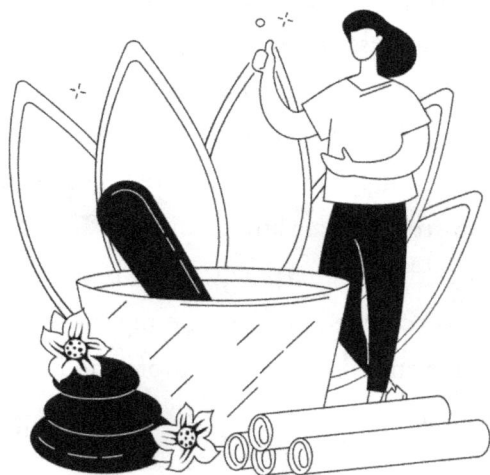

Chapter Seven
HARNESSING THE POWER OF GENETICS

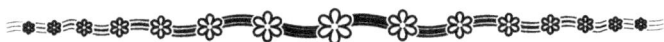

❀═❀═❀═❀═❀═❀═❀═❀═❀═❀═❀═❀═❀═❀═❀

Genetics often feels like a fixed script, but the truth is far more empowering—our DNA provides a blueprint, not a destiny. By understanding your genetic makeup, you gain a crucial edge to make informed choices that tip the scales toward a longer, healthier life. This isn't about fatalism but about recognizing how genes interact dynamically with lifestyle factors and environments, so you can intentionally shape outcomes through diet, exercise, and stress management. The emerging science of epigenetics reveals that our habits can dial genes up or down, unlocking pathways to vitality that weren't thought possible just decades ago. Harnessing this knowledge transforms longevity from passively inherited fate into an active, personalized strategy—one where you hold the reins to extend not just your years, but the quality of each one.

UNDERSTANDING YOUR GENETIC BLUEPRINT

When we talk about longevity, the conversation often turns to lifestyle choices—what we eat, how much we move, and how well we manage stress. Yet beneath these daily decisions lies a more fundamental layer: your genetic blueprint. Each of us carries a unique set of genes that influence not only our appearance and predisposition to certain diseases, but also how our bodies age over time. Understanding this blueprint can empower you to make smarter, more targeted choices that genuinely extend both lifespan and healthspan.

Genetics isn't about fate or inevitability. Instead, it's a complex map highlighting potential risks and strengths. Some people inherit variants that put them at higher risk for conditions like heart disease, diabetes, or Alzheimer's, while others carry genes associated with longevity and resilience. By getting to know your genetic makeup, you gain insight into which areas you should address proactively and where your natural advantages lie. This knowledge shifts the narrative from passively accepting the aging process to actively engaging in your health journey.

What many don't realize is that the field of genetics has evolved from simply identifying "good" or "bad" genes. It's now about understanding interactions and probabilities. That means no single gene determines your destiny; it's a network of genes, environmental factors, and behaviors working together. For example, one person might have a gene variant linked to increased inflammation, but by optimizing diet and exercise, they can often counteract or mitigate potential harm. In this way, genetics serves as a foundation for tailored strategies rather than a strict rulebook.

Many people hesitate to explore their genetics because of fear or misunderstanding. The word "genetic testing" can conjure images of medical verdicts delivered with finality—either a clean bill of health or a looming diagnosis. However, modern genetic tests focus more on probabilities and patterns, helping you pinpoint where you should invest energy rather than delivering absolute judgments. Think of your genetic report as a personalized health compass, guiding choices about nutrition, exercise, and preventive care rather than dictating a predetermined path.

Understanding your genes can also transform how you view the aging process itself. While chronological age is simple to measure, biological age, which reflects your body's functional state, can vary widely among individuals of the same birth year. Certain genetic markers correspond with slower biological aging, resilience to oxidative stress, or efficient repair mechanisms. Pinpointing these markers helps reveal how well your body is managing the wear and tear of time—and what interventions might enhance that capacity.

To truly harness the power of your genetic blueprint, however, it's essential to approach the information with context and nuance. Raw genetic data alone means little without expert interpretation. The rise of direct-to-consumer genetic tests offers convenient access, but the most effective use of this information comes from combining it with insights from healthcare professionals who understand longevity science. They can help translate the data into actionable recommendations, tailoring strategies to your distinct needs.

Consider, for instance, the genes involved in lipid metabolism. Variants in these genes may suggest an increased risk of elevated cholesterol or heart disease.

Knowing this, you can focus more rigorously on heart-healthy habits—prioritizing anti-inflammatory foods, managing weight, and maintaining regular physical activity. Conversely, if your genetic profile suggests strong antioxidant defenses, you might feel more confident in your body's ability to cope with oxidative stress, allowing for slightly different lifestyle priorities.

Another fascinating area is the role of genetics in individual responses to diet and exercise. Some people thrive on low-carbohydrate diets, while others perform best with balanced macronutrients. Similarly, genetic variants can influence how your body builds muscle, recovers from injury, or adapts to endurance training. By deciphering these clues, you can customize your nutrition and workout regimens to maximize results, reduce injury risk, and extend your vitality well into later years.

It's worth noting that genetics can also inform your approach to mental and cognitive health. Certain gene variants are linked with susceptibility to stress, mood disorders, or neurodegenerative diseases. Recognizing these predispositions isn't about resignation; it's an invitation to adopt targeted mental health practices and brain-boosting activities that support resilience and neuroplasticity. This proactive stance can be crucial for preserving cognitive function across decades.

The power of genetic knowledge truly shines when paired with a mindset of adaptability and resilience. Your genes provide a set of probabilities, not predestined outcomes. Lifestyle choices, environmental factors, and emerging technologies all play vital roles in modulating how these genetic potentials manifest. This interplay underscores a profound truth: while you can't change your inherited genes, you hold significant influence over how they express themselves.

Equally important is understanding that genetic insights extend beyond individual health. They offer a framework for familial longevity, enhancing not just your lifespan but the quality of lives across generations. Sharing genetic information with family members, when handled thoughtfully and with respect to privacy, can help guide collective health strategies. It promotes early detection, preventive action, and a culture of wellness that cascades down family lines.

For anyone pursuing longevity, there's an empowering message here: your genetic blueprint lays a foundation, not a ceiling. The knowledge you gain from your genes provides clarity on where to focus your efforts but doesn't replace the power of proactive habits, mindful living, or emotional well-being. Genetics and lifestyle aren't separate silos; they're dynamic partners in your longevity journey.

In practice, leveraging your genetic blueprint often starts with identifying key areas of concern or strength, then layering in evidence-based interventions. This approach enables a precision that generic advice can't match. Imagine being able to fine-tune your nutrition based on how your body metabolizes fats or carbohydrates, or prolonging muscle function by understanding your unique regenerative capacity. This level of personalization transforms longevity from a broad aspiration into a tangible, individualized goal.

Ultimately, embracing your genetic blueprint requires a balance of curiosity, humility, and determination. Curiosity to explore the insights your DNA holds, humility to recognize what you can't control, and determination to act on what you can influence. When these elements align, they unlock the true potential of harnessing genetics as a powerful tool in living not only longer but better.

EPIGENETICS AND LIFESTYLE MODIFICATIONS

Exploring the power of genetics has revolutionized how we think about aging and health. But genes alone don't write your fate. Epigenetics—

the suite of molecular mechanisms that regulate gene expression without altering the DNA sequence—reveals just how responsive your genetic blueprint is to your lifestyle choices. Imagine your genes as a vast library, but epigenetics acts as the librarian deciding which books get opened, read, or shut away. This fascinating interplay means your daily habits can genuinely influence how your genes perform, opening pathways to healthier, longer life.

One of the most profound insights from epigenetic research is that lifestyle modifications can prompt chemical changes—like DNA methylation and histone modification—that turn genes on or off. These are not permanent mutations; rather, they are reversible marks shaped by nutrition, stress, sleep, and physical activity. Think of it as software updates to your genetic hardware, improving how your body operates without rewriting the code itself.

Nutrition is a major player in this epigenetic symphony. Foods rich in bioactive compounds—such as polyphenols found in berries, turmeric, and green tea—have been shown to influence epigenetic markers tied to inflammation and cellular aging. In fact, the Mediterranean diet, lauded for its heart-health benefits, also supports favorable epigenetic profiles. It's

THE LONGEVITY BLUEPRINT

a clear reminder: what you eat doesn't just feed your body; it talks to your genes.

But diet is only part of the puzzle. Physical activity, particularly consistent aerobic exercise, has a remarkable impact on the epigenome. Exercise modulates gene expression related to metabolism, oxidative stress, and muscle growth. These changes promote cellular resilience, improving your body's ability to fend off age-related damage. More importantly, the benefits of altering gene expression through movement aren't limited to muscle tissue— they extend to brain health, mood regulation, and immune function.

Stress management is another critical lifestyle factor that modulates epigenetic marks. Chronic stress creates a cascade of hormonal signals that can leave lasting epigenetic imprints, particularly on genes linked with inflammation and mental health. Mindfulness practices, meditation, and adequate social support have been associated with healthier epigenetic patterns, reducing risk factors for diseases often exacerbated by stress. This demonstrates that emotional well-being and genetic health are deeply intertwined, emphasizing the importance of cultivating habits that soothe the mind.

89

Sleep, often overlooked in longevity discussions, directly affects epigenetic regulation. Poor or insufficient sleep disrupts the body's repair mechanisms and alters gene expression related to immune function and metabolism. On the flip side, quality sleep restores these epigenetic patterns, enhancing neuroplasticity and systemic renewal. Prioritizing sleep hygiene isn't just about feeling rested—it's laying the biochemical groundwork for healthier aging.

What's truly inspiring is that epigenetic changes can happen relatively quickly. Unlike static genetic mutations, which you inherit at birth, these markers adapt in response to your environment and behaviors. This opens an empowering door: your efforts in adopting healthier behaviors can literally rewrite aspects of your gene expression within weeks or months. It's not just about preventing disease but actively promoting biological youthfulness.

We also need to appreciate that epigenetics functions with a deep sense of balance. While positive lifestyle choices can enhance gene function, exposures to toxins, poor diet, sedentary habits, and chronic stress can leave negative epigenetic signatures that accelerate aging and disease risk. This understanding compels an integrated approach to wellness—one where you simultaneously promote beneficial signals and minimize harmful ones.

In practical terms, this means you don't have to overhaul your entire life overnight. Small, consistent changes—choosing whole foods over processed snacks, incorporating moderate physical activity, managing daily stress, and committing to proper sleep—compound over time to create favorable epigenetic shifts. These incremental steps translate to meaningful biological advantages that can elevate your healthspan.

Interestingly, epigenetic mechanisms also play a key role in how the body responds to caloric restriction and intermittent fasting. These popular longevity interventions don't just reduce calories; they tweak gene expression in ways that promote cellular repair, reduce inflammation, and improve metabolic efficiency. With this knowledge, it becomes clearer why certain dietary patterns championed by longevity science have such profound effects—not because they change DNA sequences, but because they recalibrate the activity of longevity-related genes.

Moreover, epigenetics underscores the importance of a personalized approach to health. Since each individual's genetic and epigenetic landscape is unique, the lifestyle modifications that optimize gene expression can vary. Genetic testing combined with epigenetic profiling presents a future where recommendations for diet, exercise, sleep, and stress management become increasingly tailored, unlocking higher potential for extending vitality in ways aligned with your biology.

It's also worth noting the intergenerational implications of epigenetics. Your lifestyle does not just affect your own gene expression but can influence the health and longevity of future generations. Epigenetic alterations in germ cells can be passed down, making your commitment to healthy habits a legacy of resilience that transcends your own lifespan.

As we harness these insights, the challenge lies in the consistent application of epigenetic-friendly behaviors amidst a world full of distractions and quick fixes. The true power of this science isn't just its novelty but in reminding us that longevity is largely within our grasp. By respecting the biochemical dialogue between lifestyle and genes, we activate a system designed for renewal, adaptation, and lasting well-being.

To integrate these ideas, consider framing your daily routines as epigenetic investments. Every meal becomes a conversation with your cells. Every moment spent moving, breathing deeply, or sleeping well is an act of genetic stewardship. This mindset transforms the pursuit of longevity from abstract science into lived experience—one where you wield your habits as tools to sculpt your biological destiny.

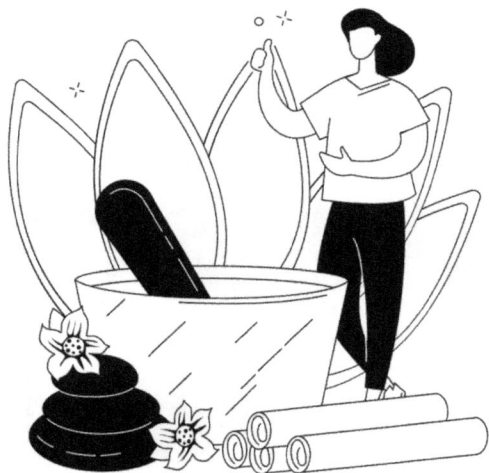

Chapter Eight
HORMONES AND AGING

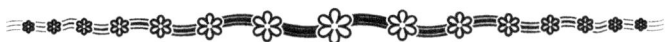

═•═❋═❋═❋═❋═❋═❋═❋═❋═❋═❋═❋═•═

A s we age, the delicate balance of hormones that governs everything from energy levels to metabolism shifts in ways that can significantly impact our healthspan, but this doesn't mean decline is inevitable; understanding how hormones influence aging unlocks powerful strategies to maintain vitality and resilience. Hormones like testosterone, estrogen, growth hormone, and cortisol play pivotal roles in cellular repair, muscle mass retention, and stress regulation, all of which can either accelerate or slow the aging process depending on their levels and interaction. By adopting lifestyle habits that support hormonal harmony—such as quality sleep, balanced nutrition, mindful stress management, and consistent physical activity—we can influence these internal chemical messengers to work in our favor rather than against us. This awareness doesn't just inspire hope; it invites intentional action, showing us that aging with strength and purpose involves more than genetics—it demands nurturing the hormone systems integral to our longevity.

KEY HORMONES THAT INFLUENCE HEALTHSPAN

Hormones act as the body's intricate chemical messengers, orchestrating a vast array of physiological processes that affect how we age. They're not just regulators of puberty or reproduction; hormones deeply shape our energy levels, immune function, tissue repair, and even mental sharpness over time. As we get older, the balance and production of key hormones shift, influencing not only lifespan but, crucially, our healthspan—the period of life spent in good health. Understanding which hormones have the most significant impact on maintaining vitality can empower anyone to apply practical strategies that support longevity with real quality of life.

The first and perhaps most well-known hormone connected to aging is **growth hormone (GH)**. Produced by the pituitary gland, GH stimulates cellular growth, regeneration, and protein synthesis. In youth, it plays a starring role in muscle and bone development, but as we age, its levels decline steadily, contributing to reduced muscle mass, thinner skin, and slower tissue repair. Low GH isn't just about outward signs; it also impacts metabolism, often leading to increased fat accumulation, especially around the abdomen, and a decrease in energy. Scientists have long debated whether supplementing GH can reverse aging effects, but it's clear that maintaining its natural balance supports physical resilience and recovery.

Closely linked to growth hormone is **insulin-like growth factor 1 (IGF-1)**, which mediates many of the growth-promoting effects. IGF-1 is a double-edged sword in longevity science. On one hand, it supports muscle maintenance, cognitive function, and heart health; on the other, excessive levels might be associated with increased risks of certain cancers. Striking the right balance is key—enough IGF-1 to sustain strength and repair without tipping the scales toward disease. Interestingly, many longevity studies correlate moderate IGF-1 levels with longer lifespans, especially when paired with healthy dietary patterns and physical activity.

Sex hormones also play a pivotal role in healthspan. Testosterone in men and estrogen and progesterone in women govern not only reproductive health but influence bone density, fat distribution, cognition, and mood regulation. The decline in these hormones, particularly after middle age, is often linked to common aging complaints: loss of libido, muscle wasting, osteoporosis, and brain fog. However, hormone replacement should be approached thoughtfully. Natural lifestyle choices can gently support healthier hormone levels without the risks associated with aggressive medical interventions. Exercise, balanced nutrition, stress management, and adequate sleep all feed into this delicate endocrine balance, underscoring that longevity isn't about chasing youthful hormone numbers but nurturing overall harmony.

The hormone **cortisol**, often called the stress hormone, deserves special attention because it directly impacts healthspan by modulating the body's response to physical and emotional stressors. Acute increases in cortisol are adaptive and help us confront challenges, but chronic elevation leads to damaging effects such as inflammation, insulin resistance, suppressed immune function, and impaired cognitive clarity. Managing cortisol through stress-reduction techniques—whether mindfulness, regular exercise, or proper rest—can protect the body and brain from accelerated aging. Hormonal health isn't only about boosting levels but also about curbing excesses that quietly erode vitality over time.

DHEA (dehydroepiandrosterone) is another hormone often called the "fountain of youth" for its association with longevity. It serves as a precursor to sex hormones and has anti-inflammatory and antioxidant properties. DHEA levels drop substantially with age, correlating with declines in immune function and energy levels. Studies suggest that individuals with higher DHEA tend to display better functional capacity in later years. However, similar to other hormones, the goal isn't to maximize DHEA indiscriminately but to support the body's ability to maintain healthy production through lifestyle, nutrition, and stress control.

The thyroid hormones—primarily **thyroxine (T4) and triiodothyronine (T3)**—are essential regulators of metabolism. As metabolism slows with aging, suboptimal thyroid function can lead to fatigue, weight gain, cold intolerance, and cognitive decline. Vital for keeping energy production efficient at the cellular level, thyroid hormones help maintain cardiovascular health and brain vitality. Even mild imbalances can undermine healthspan, yet many people go undiagnosed due to subtle symptom presentation. Routine screening and proper dietary support—such as adequate iodine and selenium intake—are simple yet effective steps to maintain optimal thyroid health for aging well.

Melatonin, commonly known as the sleep hormone, extends beyond regulating circadian rhythms. Its antioxidant capacity shields cells from damage and supports immune resilience. Aging naturally reduces melatonin production, contributing to poorer sleep quality, which in turn affects hormone production, cognitive function, and cardiovascular health. Improving sleep hygiene, managing light exposure, and promoting consistent sleep schedules can help restore beneficial melatonin cycles, amplifying the body's nightly repair processes. Melatonin's role in extending healthspan highlights how sleep and hormonal health are inseparably intertwined.

It's impossible to talk about hormones without mentioning the **insulin** system. Often maligned purely as a regulator of blood sugar, insulin's influence over cellular nutrient uptake fundamentally shapes aging trajectories. Insulin resistance, a hallmark of metabolic syndrome and type 2 diabetes, increases with age, accelerating tissue damage, inflammation, and cognitive decline. Thus, maintaining insulin sensitivity through dietary choices, physical activity, and weight management is a critical strategy for enhancing healthspan. The ongoing challenge is to preserve this system's delicate balance since both excess and deficiency can have profound health effects.

All these hormones interact within a complex network, meaning optimal healthspan depends on balance rather than isolated hormone levels. This interconnectedness explains why holistic approaches to longevity—which focus on diet, exercise, sleep, and stress reduction—align with the natural rhythms of the endocrine system. The endocrine glands don't operate in silos; instead, they communicate dynamically, responding to environmental inputs and lifestyle choices in ways that either promote resilience or accelerate decline.

Amid the popular fascination with hormone replacement therapies, it's crucial to recognize that simply supplementing hormones isn't a guaranteed path to longer life or better healthspan. Hormones serve as signals rather than cures by themselves. The goal isn't to fight aging by trying to recapture adolescent hormone surges but to support the body's own ability to regulate and produce hormones efficiently. That means prioritizing nutrition that feeds hormone production, exercising regularly to stimulate hormonal pathways, managing stress to keep hormones like cortisol in check, and maintaining restful sleep patterns to support melatonin and growth hormone cycles.

In practice, attention to these "key" hormones becomes a guide for lifestyle decisions that enhance overall vitality. They offer a window into underlying physiological health and pinpoint areas where small shifts can yield significant improvements. By tuning into how hormones impact energy, recovery, mood, and immunity, health-conscious individuals can make informed choices that support not only longer life but better years filled with vigor and purpose.

In sum, hormones represent a powerful axis through which aging can be modulated. Recognizing their roles, respecting their balance, and adopting daily habits that nurture their function equips everyone with a practical roadmap to extend healthspan. The promise lies not in chasing youthful hormone peaks but in cultivating sustainable, balanced hormonal health that fuels a vibrant, thriving life well into advanced years.

NATURAL WAYS TO SUPPORT HORMONAL BALANCE

As we journey through life, our hormones play a pivotal role in shaping both our physical health and emotional well-being. Yet, with aging, this delicate balance often shifts, leading many to experience symptoms like fatigue, weight gain, mood swings, and decreased vitality. Supporting hormonal balance naturally is a cornerstone of maintaining healthspan— the period of life spent in good health—without relying on synthetic interventions or quick fixes. The good news is that the body has an incredible capacity to regulate itself, especially when given the right tools and environment.

One of the foundational approaches to nurturing hormonal harmony is through diet. Hormones are synthesized from nutrients, and inadequate or excessive intake can create ripple effects throughout the endocrine system. Incorporating whole, nutrient-dense foods supplies the body with essential building blocks such as healthy fats, vitamins, and minerals that serve as precursors or cofactors for hormone production. For instance, omega-3 fatty acids, abundant in fatty fish, flaxseeds, and walnuts, support the production of anti-inflammatory hormones that protect cells from damage. Equally important are micronutrients like zinc and magnesium, which have been shown to assist in regulating insulin, cortisol, and sex hormones.

But it's not just about what you eat; how you eat matters too. Avoiding large spikes and dips in blood sugar is a simple yet powerful way to prevent hormonal upheaval. Frequent consumption of refined sugars and processed grains forces the pancreas to release insulin repeatedly, which can lead to insulin resistance over time—a key driver of aging and chronic disease. Stabilizing blood sugar through balanced meals helps keep insulin and other metabolic hormones in check, indirectly easing the workload on adrenal and thyroid glands.

Physical movement is another vital ally in this quest. Exercise acts as a natural hormone modulator, stimulating the release of endorphins, regulating insulin sensitivity, and influencing growth hormone and testosterone levels. Importantly, the type and intensity of exercise can determine its effects on hormones. Strength training, for example, promotes anabolic hormones that preserve muscle mass and bone density, while moderate aerobic exercise reduces cortisol, the stress hormone that in excess can wreak havoc on metabolic health. Yet, it's crucial to avoid overtraining, which can tip the balance toward chronic stress and hormonal exhaustion.

Sleep deserves special emphasis here because it's when the body carries out much of its restorative hormone production. Growth hormone surges primarily during deep sleep phases, facilitating tissue repair and cellular regeneration. Melatonin, the hormone that regulates our sleep-wake cycle, also acts as an antioxidant, defending cells against age-related damage. Poor sleep disrupts these processes and leads to elevated cortisol, impaired glucose metabolism, and imbalance in sex hormones like estrogen and testosterone—it's no surprise that sleep deprivation ages us prematurely. Strategies like maintaining a consistent bedtime, limiting screen exposure before sleep, and creating a dark, cool resting environment foster the optimal hormonal milieu for recovery.

Stress management cannot be overstated when it comes to hormonal health. Chronic psychological and physiological stress elevate cortisol production, which in turn suppresses the immune system, inhibits insulin function, and alters reproductive hormones. Mindfulness practices, meditation, deep breathing, and even simple acts of spending time in nature have been proven to lower stress markers. These activities influence the hypothalamic-pituitary-adrenal axis, resetting the body's stress response and allowing hormones to operate within balanced parameters. Over time, cultivating resilience to stress can profoundly support longevity by preserving both hormonal and cellular integrity.

Another natural avenue is the strategic use of botanicals and adaptogens—plants that have traditionally been used to enhance the body's response to stress and support hormonal regulation. Ashwagandha, rhodiola, and holy basil are just a few examples known for their ability to modulate cortisol levels, improve energy, and promote mental clarity. While these herbs complement a healthy lifestyle, they're best used with awareness and care, ideally under the guidance of a healthcare provider familiar with natural medicine, especially because each individual's hormonal landscape is unique.

Hydration may seem mundane, but proper water intake is essential for hormone transport and function. Dehydration can increase the production of vasopressin, a hormone that helps regulate fluid balance but also signals the release of stress hormones.

Drinking enough water throughout the day supports cellular communication and waste removal, ensuring hormones reach their target tissues efficiently. Pairing hydration with mineral-rich water enhances this effect further, supplying electrolytes crucial for endocrine health.

Beyond individual lifestyle choices, environmental factors also influence hormonal balance. Minimizing exposure to endocrine disruptors found in plastics, pesticides, and some personal care products reduces the burden on the endocrine system. These chemicals can mimic or block natural hormones, confusing your body's signaling systems and accelerating age-related decline. Using natural, non-toxic products and advocating for clean environments create a protective barrier for hormonal health, aligning well with broader goals of longevity and vitality.

Finally, cultivating social connections and fostering emotional well-being cannot be overlooked as a natural way to support hormones. Positive relationships stimulate oxytocin, the "bonding hormone," which counters stress and supports heart health. Feeling supported and engaged contributes to lower cortisol levels and balanced reproductive hormones. In contrast, social isolation and loneliness have been linked to increased risk of hormonal dysregulation and inflammation. Building and nurturing relationships is a vital piece of the hormonal health puzzle, underscoring how deeply connected our biology is with our environment and lifestyle.

In essence, harmonizing hormones naturally is about creating balance—a synergy between what we consume, how we move, rest, handle stress, and relate to others. It recognizes the power of small, consistent choices over time that, when compounded, foster an internal environment where hormones can thrive. As we age, these choices become even more critical, providing a strong foundation for prolonged healthspan and the kind of vibrant life we aspire to live. Your hormones are not simply markers of aging; they are dynamic messengers that respond to the world you build for yourself every day. Embrace this understanding and let it inspire a holistic approach that supports you, not just to live longer, but to live fuller.

Chapter Nine
IMMUNE SYSTEM AND LONGEVITY

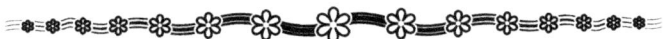

Our immune system isn't just about fighting off colds or infections—it's a cornerstone of lasting health and lifespan. When it functions well, it keeps chronic inflammation in check, supports tissue repair, and helps the body adapt to stresses that would otherwise accelerate aging. Strengthening immune resilience means adopting habits that consistently nourish and challenge this vital defense network without overwhelming it. This includes lifestyle choices that promote balance, like quality nutrition, moderate exercise, and stress management, which collectively fortify immune responses and dampen destructive inflammation. Ultimately, a robust immune system acts as a guardian of longevity by maintaining cellular integrity and preventing the diseases that shorten life, making it an essential focus for anyone serious about living not just longer, but healthier years

ENHANCING IMMUNE RESILIENCE

The immune system isn't just our body's defense mechanism against infections—it's a critical pillar supporting longevity and overall vitality. As we age, the immune system undergoes a natural decline known as immunosenescence, which leaves us more vulnerable to illnesses and diminishes our ability to recover. Enhancing immune resilience isn't about chasing an elusive cure; it's about adopting practical, science-backed strategies that strengthen our body's capacity to fend off threats and maintain balance.

Immune resilience refers to the ability of the immune system to respond efficiently to challenges while avoiding harmful overreactions like chronic inflammation. When this balance is struck, it creates an environment where cellular repair processes thrive, and the body can better resist age-related diseases. Strengthening immune resilience sets the stage for not only longer life but a higher quality of life—a life where healthspan matches lifespan.

One of the foundational approaches to boosting immune function involves nurturing your body's natural defenses through lifestyle choices that support both innate and adaptive immunity. This isn't about quick fixes or supplements alone; it requires consistent, holistic changes that improve how your immune cells originate, mature, and coordinate responses.

Physical activity plays an indispensable role here. Moderate, regular exercise has been shown to stimulate immune surveillance by enhancing circulation, which helps immune cells patrol the body more effectively. It reduces inflammation, partly by lowering visceral fat stores that produce pro-inflammatory compounds. However, the key is balance: excessive or intense training without adequate recovery can actually suppress immune function, so it's essential to find an exercise routine that challenges but doesn't overwhelm your system.

Sleep is often underestimated but holds a critical position in immune health. During deep sleep stages, the body releases cytokines, which are proteins that help regulate immune responses and inflammation. Chronic sleep deprivation disrupts this process, weakening defenses and increasing susceptibility to infections. Aiming for consistent, restorative sleep lays a powerful foundation for maintaining immune resilience through the years.

The intersection of stress and immunity is another critical factor. Chronic psychological stress triggers prolonged release of cortisol and other stress hormones that, over time, impair immune cell function. Techniques like mindfulness meditation, controlled breathing, and even simple acts like spending time in nature can significantly reduce stress hormones and recalibrate immune responses. Developing stress management rituals isn't just about mental well-being—it's a direct investment in your immune durability.

Nutrition also shapes immune competence. While comprehensive dietary insights are covered elsewhere, the overall narrative here is that a nutrient-dense diet rich in antioxidants, vitamins, and minerals forms the biochemical scaffolding for immune cells. Nutrients such as vitamin D, zinc, and omega-3 fatty acids support various aspects of immune function, from cell signaling to inflammation control. Equally important is limiting excess sugar and processed foods that can promote systemic inflammation and weaken immunity.

Hydration and gut health also interlink tightly with immune defense. The gut houses nearly 70 percent of immune cells, acting as a critical battleground where balance determines outcomes. While more detailed discussion follows in other sections, simple daily habits—like consuming fiber-rich foods that nurture beneficial gut microbes and drinking adequate water—create an environment for a healthy barrier against pathogens and facilitate immune training.

Another piece of immune resilience lies in embracing responsible exposure to the world around us. Over-sanitization might seem protective, but evidence suggests that a certain amount of microbial interaction is essential for calibrating and educating the immune system. This principle, sometimes called the "hygiene hypothesis," highlights why getting outside, gardening, or even having pets can contribute to a better-regulated immune response. Natural environments introduce diverse microorganisms that strengthen immune tolerance and resilience.

Age brings inevitable shifts in immune characteristics, yet how we approach these changes defines whether immunity stagnates or adapts.

Vaccination remains a crucial tool in sustaining immune defense, especially in older adults. Staying up to date with recommended vaccines doesn't just reduce the risk of serious diseases but also stimulates immune memory, reinforcing the system's ability to recognize and respond efficiently.

Emerging science reveals fascinating avenues to enhance immune function by tapping into the body's regenerative capacity. Interventions such as intermittent fasting have shown promise in promoting immune cell renewal by triggering autophagy, a natural process that clears out damaged cells and supports the generation of new immune cells. While not a universal prescription, carefully implemented fasting protocols under professional supervision can boost immune surveillance and reduce chronic inflammation.

Maintaining social connections isn't just emotionally fulfilling, it also bolsters immune resilience. Meaningful relationships and community support buffer against stress-induced immune suppression. Loneliness and social isolation have been linked to increased inflammatory markers and poorer immune responses. Cultivating authentic social bonds acts as a protective factor that enhances vitality and longevity.

While genetics influence how our immune system functions, lifestyle choices vastly impact its trajectory. Epigenetic changes—those modifications in gene expression influenced by our environment and behaviors—can either weaken or strengthen immune responses. This means habit shifts undertaken today have the power to rewrite immune aging patterns tomorrow.

Ultimately, enhancing immune resilience requires an integrated approach. There is no single magic bullet, but the synergy of nutritious foods, physical movement, proper rest, stress regulation, meaningful social ties, and smart medical care builds a fortress against age-related immune decline. It's about equipping the body's natural defenses to operate at their peak for as long as possible.

Longevity isn't solely about adding years to life; it's about adding life to years. Strengthening immune resilience fuels that mission by reducing vulnerability and empowering your body to heal, adapt, and thrive. These practical steps—often simple yet profoundly impactful—can transform how your immune system supports every facet of your well-being as you age.

THE GUT MICROBIOME'S ROLE IN IMMUNE HEALTH

When it comes to longevity, few factors are as quietly powerful as the state of your gut microbiome. This bustling community of trillions of bacteria, viruses, fungi, and other microorganisms plays an essential role far beyond digestion. In fact, the gut microbiome is a critical player in shaping immune health, which in turn affects your body's ability to stay resilient against diseases and maintain vitality throughout life.

Imagine your gut as a complex ecosystem where beneficial microbes live in harmony with your body. These microbes interact directly with immune cells and influence how immune responses are triggered and regulated. A balanced microbiome doesn't just defend you well against infection; it helps keep chronic inflammation in check, which is one of the biggest contributors to aging and age-related diseases.

Research now reveals that roughly 70-80% of the immune system resides in or around the gut. This means what happens inside your digestive tract profoundly affects systemic immunity. The gut lining acts as a frontline barrier, with microbes helping to fortify this boundary and prevent harmful pathogens from crossing into the bloodstream. Microbes also train immune cells to differentiate between harmless and harmful invaders, reducing the risk of autoimmune reactions where the body turns against itself.

Yet, not all microbes are beneficial—some can provoke inflammation and weaken immune defenses. This imbalance, often called dysbiosis, has been linked to numerous chronic conditions, from allergies and asthma to autoimmune diseases and metabolic disorders. For anyone focused on living longer and healthier, nurturing a balanced gut microbiome becomes a targeted approach to supporting immune resilience throughout the aging process.

One of the most exciting aspects of gut-immune interaction lies in the microbial production of short-chain fatty acids (SCFAs), such as butyrate, propionate, and acetate. These compounds arise when friendly bacteria ferment dietary fiber, and they have far-reaching effects on immune function. SCFAs promote the development of regulatory T cells, which are vital for keeping inflammatory responses under control. They also support the integrity of the gut barrier, preventing leaky gut syndrome—a condition implicated in chronic inflammation and many degenerative diseases.

Now, think about how diet plays a role here. Poor dietary choices can starve beneficial microbes, leading to decreased SCFA production and a weakened gut barrier. Conversely, a diet rich in diverse plant fibers, fermented foods, and polyphenols feeds the microbial community, fostering an environment that encourages immune balance and long-term health.

It's tempting to view the immune system as an isolated defense unit, but that's just not how it works. The gut microbiome acts as a communication hub between the environment and the body's defenses. When this communication flows smoothly, immune responses are swift but measured. When disrupted, the immune system may either overreact, causing inflammation and tissue damage, or underperform, leaving you vulnerable to infections.

- **Supporting microbial diversity:** A diverse microbiome has been consistently linked to stronger immunity and better health outcomes. Diversity is a natural defense mechanism, preventing dominance by harmful species and ensuring immune responses are well-coordinated.

- **Maintaining gut barrier integrity:** The gut lining is more than just a physical barrier. It actively signals to immune cells and influences the threshold at

THE LONGEVITY BLUEPRINT

which responses are activated. Strengthening this barrier limits systemic inflammation and protects against pathogens.

- **Regulating inflammation:** Chronic low-grade inflammation accelerates aging and underpins many diseases. The microbiome's ability to modulate inflammation through metabolites and immune education is a crucial longevity mechanism.

Beyond diet, lifestyle factors including stress, sleep patterns, and physical activity have profound effects on the gut microbiota and, by extension, immune health. Chronic stress, for example, can disrupt microbial balance and increase intestinal permeability. Meanwhile, regular exercise has been shown to enhance microbial diversity and support immune homeostasis. Sleep deprivation similarly alters gut bacteria composition and impairs immune surveillance, highlighting how interconnected these systems truly are.

In the quest for a longer, healthier life, this growing understanding of the gut-immune axis invites practical interventions that anyone can adopt. Probiotic and prebiotic therapies, while still an area of active research, offer potential ways to jumpstart or

119

maintain a healthy microbial environment. But more importantly, sustainable lifestyle changes that promote microbial diversity and barrier health should be the cornerstone of any longevity strategy. Eating whole foods rich in fiber, engaging in regular physical activity, managing stress effectively, and prioritizing sleep are proven ways to cultivate a resilient microbiome and, by extension, a robust immune system.

The implications for longevity are profound. Aging often brings a decline in immune function, referred to as immunosenescence, which increases susceptibility to infections, cancer, and chronic inflammation. However, by preserving a balanced gut microbiome, it's possible to slow this decline, ensuring your immune system remains responsive but not reactive. This balanced immune state can reduce the risk of chronic diseases, improve recovery from illness, and even enhance vaccine responses in older adults.

What does this mean in practical terms? It means recognizing that your gut health isn't just about comfort or digestion—it's a foundational pillar for lifelong resilience. Taking care of your microbiome is investing in your biological toolkit for combating the stresses and strains that come with aging. This approach is empowering, putting control over immune function and longevity directly in your hands through everyday choices.

Emerging research continues to uncover novel ways that gut microbes influence immune cells far beyond the gut itself, including effects on liver function, brain inflammation, and systemic metabolic health. These insights underscore the microbiome as a systemic regulator, not a passive passenger. As the science unfolds, new therapies targeting the gut-immune axis may revolutionize how we approach aging and disease prevention.

Until then, the best strategy is to nurture your gut ecosystem consistently. Simple habits like eating fermented foods—kimchi, yogurt, sauerkraut—and increasing fiber-rich vegetables can transform your microbial landscape. Avoiding unnecessary antibiotics, reducing processed foods, and maintaining a healthy stress-sleep-exercise balance will keep your immune system primed for the challenges of aging.

The story of the gut microbiome's role in immune health perfectly illustrates a larger truth about longevity: lasting health is not about silver-bullet solutions but about nurturing complex systems that work together harmoniously. Your immune system thrives when your gut ecosystem flourishes, and by prioritizing this connection, you lay a foundation for both a longer life and a better quality of life.

Chapter Ten
CUTTING-EDGE LONGEVITY TECHNOLOGIES

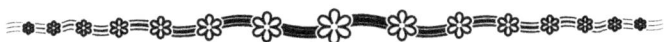

Advancements in longevity science have ushered in a new era where technology isn't just about convenience—it's actively reshaping how we age and how long we live. From gene editing tools that promise to correct age-related damage at its source to novel drug therapies targeting cellular rejuvenation, these innovations push the boundaries of what was once thought possible. Yet, it's not just the science that's evolving; accessibility and ethical questions are shaping how these technologies will integrate into daily life, ensuring they serve more than just a select few. Embracing these breakthroughs with discernment can empower us to enhance not only lifespan but, crucially, healthspan—giving every extra year vibrant meaning rather than mere existence.

EMERGING THERAPIES AND INTERVENTIONS

The landscape of longevity science has evolved far beyond the traditional advice of diet and exercise. Today, emerging therapies and interventions hold unprecedented promise for extending not only lifespan but, crucially, healthspan—the years we spend feeling vibrant and capable. These innovations blend cutting-edge biotechnology with a deeper understanding of the aging process, promising to rewrite what it means to grow older. For those aiming to embrace a longer, healthier life, it's essential to stay informed about these developments, discerning between hype and genuinely transformative approaches.

At the forefront of these emerging therapies are cellular and molecular techniques designed to address one of aging's most profound drivers: the gradual decline in cellular function. Regenerative medicine, particularly stem cell therapy, has garnered significant attention. Stem cells' ability to differentiate into various cell types and repair damaged tissues suggests a powerful avenue to combat degeneration. Already, clinical trials are underway targeting age-related conditions such as osteoarthritis and cardiovascular disease, demonstrating encouraging results. The potential here is not merely to treat symptoms but to restore youthful function at the cellular level.

But regenerative therapies extend beyond stem cells. The notion of cellular reprogramming, where mature cells are nudged back into a more youthful state, is gaining traction. This approach bypasses some of the limitations of stem cells by rejuvenating existing tissue rather than replacing it. Early research indicates that reprogramming factors might one day help repair damage from chronic diseases or perhaps even slow the clock of aging itself. Though still in nascent stages, the trajectory is clear: harnessing the body's own biological machinery to maintain or restore vitality.

Another breakthrough comes from the realm of senolytics—compounds designed to target and eliminate senescent cells. These cells, often referred to as "zombie cells," accumulate with age and contribute to inflammation and tissue dysfunction. Removing them has shown promising results in animal studies, improving physical function and extending lifespan. Senolytic therapies represent a practical intervention that targets a root cause of aging rather than fragmented symptoms, paving the way for more comprehensive strategies to maintain healthspan.

Closely linked is the exploration of mitochondrial health. Mitochondria, often dubbed the powerhouse of the cell, play a vital role in energy production and metabolic regulation. As we age, mitochondrial function tends to decline, leading to less efficient energy use and increased oxidative stress. Advances in therapies targeting mitochondrial repair or enhancement could mitigate this decline, improving overall cellular resilience. Techniques such as mitochondrial transfer or specialized supplements that support mitochondrial biogenesis are already being tested, reflecting a shift towards addressing aging at its energetic foundation.

The role of the immune system in longevity cannot be overstated, and emerging immunotherapies continue to reshape how we think about aging and disease prevention. Chronic low-grade inflammation, or "inflammaging," underpins many age-related diseases. Novel interventions aimed at modulating immune responses seek to reduce this burden while maintaining the immune system's capacity to fight infections and malignancies. Researchers are investigating vaccines, immune checkpoint modulators, and microbiome-targeted therapies as means to recalibrate immune health in aging populations. This is a dynamic field with considerable potential to improve both lifespan and life quality.

Gene editing technologies, particularly CRISPR-Cas9, have revolutionized the possibilities for precision interventions in aging. The ability to modify or correct genetic elements implicated in age-related decline offers a tantalizing prospect. While widespread clinical application is still on the horizon, early studies show promise in tackling genetic diseases and enhancing cellular repair mechanisms. This rapidly advancing field might one day enable us to "fix" the genetic quirks that accelerate aging, reducing vulnerabilities across multiple organ systems. Ethical considerations remain paramount, but the science is advancing steadily towards targeted, safe applications.

Alongside these biological interventions, bioelectronic medicine is emerging as a novel frontier. Devices that use electrical stimulation to optimize neurochemical signaling and regulate physiological systems can positively influence aging processes. For example, vagus nerve stimulation has shown potential in reducing inflammation and improving mood and cognitive function—factors deeply tied to longevity.

These technologies provide non-invasive, adjunctive options that complement more traditional therapies and lifestyle changes, giving individuals new tools to maintain their health as they age.

Importantly, these therapies and interventions don't exist in isolation. The future of longevity lies in integrated approaches that combine multiple modalities to address the complex, multifactorial nature of aging. Bioinformatics and AI-driven diagnostics enable highly personalized treatment plans, optimizing when and how to apply these emerging interventions. This personalized strategy ensures interventions target the most relevant pathways for each individual, maximizing benefits and minimizing risks.

All these advances underscore a new paradigm— aging as a malleable process rather than an inevitable decline. This shift empowers health-conscious individuals not just to accept their biological fate but to actively participate in shaping their aging trajectory. However, it's crucial to approach these emerging therapies with a discerning eye. While promising, many are still in experimental phases, and ongoing research will define their safety and efficacy over time.

The drive towards practical application means that many of these therapies could become accessible in the coming years. For those serious about longevity, staying informed and partnering with knowledgeable healthcare providers will make a significant difference. Emerging therapies represent potential game-changers, capable of transforming how we age if adopted wisely and integrated with foundational health practices covered earlier in this book.

Embracing these innovations also calls for a mindful balance. Cutting-edge technologies should complement—not replace—the core principles of nutrition, exercise, sleep, and stress management. After all, no therapy can outpace the benefits of living well daily. The real power lies in harmonizing time-tested strategies with breakthroughs, forging a longevity blueprint that is both scientifically grounded and practically attainable.

In summary, emerging therapies and interventions are redefining what's possible for extending healthspan. From cellular rejuvenation to immune modulation, from gene editing to bioelectronic medicine, these advances offer exciting opportunities. They invite us to envision a future where aging is less about decline and more about sustained vitality. For those ready to seize these possibilities, the journey toward a longer, healthier life is entering a bold new chapter—with science and innovation lighting the way.

ETHICAL CONSIDERATIONS AND ACCESSIBILITY

As longevity research and technology advance at an unprecedented pace, the conversation about ethics and accessibility becomes not just necessary but urgent. Cutting-edge interventions like gene editing, stem cell therapies, and advanced diagnostics hold incredible promise for extending human lifespan and improving quality of life. Yet, this promise comes with profound ethical challenges that threaten to undermine the very goals these technologies aspire to achieve.

One of the most pressing ethical concerns revolves around equity. Innovations in longevity are often expensive and complex, typically available first to wealthy individuals or those living in developed countries with advanced healthcare infrastructures. This unequal access risks creating a divide where extended life and improved healthspan become privileges rather than rights. What good is a breakthrough therapy if it remains out of reach for the majority? For those who champion longevity, this isn't merely a question of fairness—it's a call to action. We have to think critically about how these technologies can become broadly accessible without sacrificing innovation or quality.

Inclusion and representation also demand attention. Scientific research historically has suffered from biases related to gender, race, socioeconomic status, and geographic location. This can lead to treatments and technologies that are less effective for certain populations, reinforcing existing disparities in health outcomes. Ethical longevity science calls for diverse clinical trials and inclusive research practices so that breakthroughs benefit everyone, not just a select demographic. Broad inclusivity not only improves efficacy but fosters trust—a crucial element for public acceptance and adoption.

Privacy is another cornerstone of ethical considerations in modern longevity efforts. Many of these technologies rely heavily on personal biological data—genetic sequences, metabolic profiles, detailed health records—to tailor interventions. While personalized medicine can revolutionize health outcomes, it raises questions about data security and consent. Users must be assured their information won't be exploited, sold, or mishandled. Transparency about how data is used and protected must be non-negotiable, or people risk losing trust in the very tools designed to help them live longer, healthier lives.

Moreover, the inevitable uncertainty surrounding long-term effects of these novel technologies points to the importance of precaution. While many longevity interventions are grounded in promising science, we're still understanding their full impact. Therapies manipulating fundamental biological pathways could have unintended consequences, both for individuals and for society at large. Rigorous, ongoing ethical review is essential, balancing eagerness to innovate with the caution necessary to protect human well-being. That balance is a fine line but crucial for advancing responsible science.

Accessibility ties directly into social and economic dimensions, too. If longevity-enhancing technologies stay confined to high-end clinics or require lifelong costly treatments, the gap between who benefits and who doesn't will widen. There's a genuine risk of reinforcing societal inequities, where the wealthiest not only have longer lives but better overall health, leaving others behind. Advocates in the field must push for policies that support universal access and insurance coverage, ensuring breakthroughs do not become tools of exclusion.

Community engagement plays a critical role in shaping ethical deployment of these technologies. Genuine dialogue with diverse publics can illuminate concerns that scientists and policymakers might overlook. Listening to varied voices allows for the creation of regulations and guidelines that balance innovation with respect for cultural values and individual autonomy. Enhanced education about both the potentials and limits of longevity technologies empowers people to make informed choices without being misled by hype or fear.

Another angle often missed in public discourse is the environmental footprint of longevity medicine. Scalable manufacture and delivery of these advanced therapies can consume significant resources, from raw materials to energy. As we aspire to longer, healthier lives, integrating sustainability into the equation is paramount. Ethics must extend beyond the patient to consider planetary health, acknowledging that any path forward should minimize harm to ecosystems upon which we all depend.

We also have to confront the ethical question of prioritization. Healthcare systems everywhere operate under resource constraints. Should immense funding be directed toward longevity interventions that primarily benefit the elderly, or should investment focus on preventative care and improving lifespan across entire populations? This is not an either-or situation, but it underscores the importance of careful resource allocation that maximizes public good while respecting individual choice.

Importantly, ethical reflection must go hand in hand with practical steps toward inclusivity. Lowering costs, simplifying delivery methods, and creating scalable solutions are essential strategies. Public-private partnerships and innovation in healthcare policy can drive these reforms. Encouraging open science and data sharing accelerates collective progress and democratizes knowledge, preventing monopolies over life-extending technologies.

At its core, accessibility is about empowerment. It means equipping people with the knowledge, tools, and opportunities to participate actively in their longevity journey. Health literacy initiatives and culturally sensitive communication can dismantle barriers often imposed by health disparities. Ensuring no one is left behind reflects the true spirit of longevity's promise— not just more years, but better years, shared equitably across society.

The journey toward extending human lifespan is as much about values as it is about science. Cutting-edge longevity technologies hold enormous transformative potential, but we must remain vigilant to the ethical implications that come with such power. With thoughtful dialogue, inclusive research, and deliberate policy, we can steer these innovations toward becoming catalysts for a healthier, fairer future—one where longevity truly means a life well-lived by all.

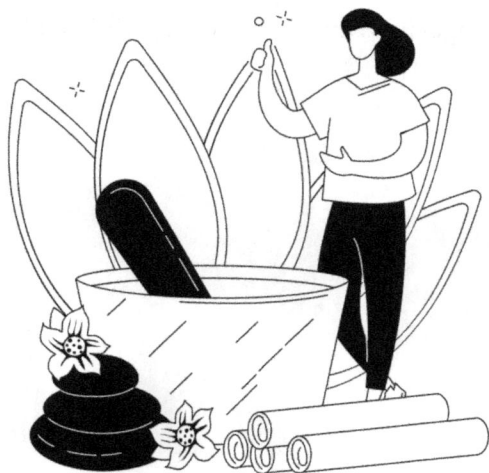

Chapter Eleven
SOCIAL CONNECTIONS AND LIFESPAN

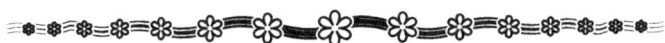

The power of social connections goes far beyond mere companionship; it deeply influences how long and how well we live. People who cultivate meaningful relationships and feel genuinely supported by their communities tend to exhibit lower risks of chronic illnesses, reduced inflammation, and even stronger immune responses. These ties not only provide emotional resilience during challenging times but also encourage healthier behaviors, from better diet choices to increased physical activity. Longevity isn't just about genes or diet—it's about belonging, purposeful interaction, and the shared human experience that fuels motivation and mental wellbeing. To truly extend your lifespan and enrich your quality of life, prioritize fostering authentic bonds; they act as a foundational pillar that supports every other longevity strategy you adopt.

THE LONGEVITY BENEFITS OF COMMUNITY

Humans are inherently social creatures. The connections we forge don't just enrich our everyday experiences—they play a critical role in how long and well we live. Community, in its many forms, serves as a powerful foundation for longevity. It provides support, reduces stress, and fosters a sense of belonging that directly influences both physical and mental health. In fact, the quality of our social ties often predicts lifespan better than many traditional risk factors like smoking, obesity, or sedentary behavior.

The impact of community on longevity is not merely about having people around but about meaningful, reciprocal relationships that cultivate trust and emotional safety. When people feel deeply connected, their bodies respond positively. The stress hormone cortisol—linked to inflammation and accelerated aging—is typically lower in individuals who experience strong social support. Simultaneously, levels of oxytocin, sometimes called the 'bonding hormone,' increase, promoting healing and reducing cardiovascular risks. These physiological benefits create an ideal internal environment that favors repair processes and enhances resilience to illness.

Living in a supportive community encourages healthier behaviors as well. People surrounded by friends and family who care tend to adopt better habits. Whether it's getting regular exercise, eating more fruits and vegetables, or attending check-ups, the positive influence of close social circles can serve as motivation and accountability. Community acts as both a safety net and a catalyst for thriving, especially when life's challenges arise. It's no coincidence that social isolation and loneliness have been identified as major public health concerns linked to higher mortality rates worldwide.

Beyond individual behaviors, community engagement nurtures purpose and meaning—two elements strongly tied to longevity. When you belong to a group, whether it's a local club, faith-based organization, or volunteer network, you have roles to play and contributions to make. This sense of purpose shifts attention away from the self and toward something bigger, reducing feelings of emptiness and depression that often accompany isolation. The motivation to serve, support, and connect sustains emotional vitality throughout the years.

Another key factor is the mental stimulation that emerges from social interaction. Conversation, collaboration, and even friendly debate challenge cognitive function and promote neuroplasticity, the brain's ability to adapt and grow new neural pathways. Keeping your mind active in a social setting nourishes cognitive longevity by delaying cognitive decline and lowering the risk of dementia. Community creates natural opportunities for mental engagement—which can feel effortless compared to structured brain-training exercises—and that continuous stimulation pays dividends as we age.

Interestingly, communities also contribute to resilience against trauma and chronic illness. When health setbacks occur, having people who provide emotional support, assist with treatment adherence, or simply offer companionship lightens the burden. Research shows that patients with robust social networks recover more quickly and have better outcomes across diverse conditions, from heart attacks to cancer. This support improves adherence to medication, promotes healthy lifestyle modifications, and buffers the psychological distress that often accompanies serious illness.

Physical safety is another practical dimension of community that influences longevity. Neighbors looking out for one another, shared vigilance, and collective resources create environments where older adults, in particular, can age in place safely. Moreover, community-based programs, such as walking groups or group exercise classes, create additional layers of motivation and infrastructure for healthy habits. This prevents or delays decline that could lead to premature institutionalization or disability.

The science behind these observations continues to grow stronger. Epidemiological studies consistently find that social integration—measured by the number and quality of relationships—is one of the most reliable predictors of lifespan. Meta-analyses reveal that people with strong social ties enjoy a 50% greater chance of survival over periods of time than those without such connections. These effects remain significant even after controlling for socioeconomic status, lifestyle factors, and pre-existing conditions. In other words, community benefits operate independently and synergistically with other longevity practices.

A crucial step in harnessing the longevity benefits of community is intention. It's not enough to passively attend social gatherings or maintain superficial contacts. Developing deep, trusting, and supportive relationships requires effort—regular communication, empathy, and shared experiences. Setting priorities that include nurturing existing bonds while also cultivating new ones lays the groundwork for lasting impact. Just like physical exercise strengthens muscles, social engagement strengthens the networks that support your health.

For those who feel socially disconnected, building community might start with small changes. Joining interest-based groups, attending local events, or volunteering in causes you care about are excellent starting points. Technology offers additional ways to connect meaningfully, but it's essential to balance online interactions with face-to-face experiences. The emotional richness found in physical presence and shared activities offers unmatched benefits for health and longevity.

As the years advance, community becomes even more vital. Social circles naturally shrink due to mobility challenges, losses, or retirement. This makes proactive engagement crucial to avoid isolation's detrimental effects. Friends and neighbors who check in regularly, support systems that offer companionship, and intergenerational connections keep life vibrant and full of purpose. The wisdom and stories exchanged within communities become treasures that not only enrich the individual but also fortify the collective.

In the quest for a longer, healthier life, embracing community is not merely a pleasant addition—it's a fundamental pillar. Physical health, mental well-being, and emotional resilience are all intertwined with the friendships, relationships, and social roles we cultivate. The benefits ripple outward, creating a positive cascade that supports longevity on multiple levels. Building and maintaining authentic connections isn't just about living longer; it's about enriching every day with the vitality and meaning that make life worth living.

Unlocking the full potential of community in your life means prioritizing it with the same commitment you give to nutrition, exercise, or sleep. Set time aside to nurture your relationships, be present in shared moments, and seek out new social opportunities that resonate with your values. The rewards extend far beyond enjoyment—they activate biological processes that keep your body youthful and your mind sharp. In this way, community acts as a powerful prescription for longevity, one that's accessible, sustainable, and deeply human.

NURTURING RELATIONSHIPS FOR BETTER HEALTH OUTCOMES

Human beings are inherently social creatures. The quality of our relationships plays a profound role in shaping not only our emotional wellbeing but also our physical health. Numerous studies have shown that fostering close, supportive connections can be as vital to our lifespan as diet or exercise. Building and maintaining these bonds isn't just about feeling good emotionally—it's about laying the foundation for a longer, healthier life.

When people feel connected, their bodies often respond in remarkable ways. Stress levels tend to drop, inflammation eases, and immune systems strengthen. On the other hand, social isolation and loneliness can have the opposite effect—leading to heightened risks of cardiovascular disease, weakened immunity, and even cognitive decline. This isn't just correlation; there's mounting evidence that the absence of nurturing relationships actively accelerates biological aging. The influence of social bonds on health is a powerful reminder that longevity isn't just built in the gym or the kitchen, but in the circles we keep day by day.

One compelling reason nurturing close relationships improves health outcomes lies in the way they help us manage stress. Chronic stress floods the body with cortisol and other hormones that, if left unchecked, can damage cells and tissues over time. When life throws curveballs—and it always does—supportive friends or family cushion the blow. A trusted confidant validates emotions, provides perspective, and encourages healthy coping mechanisms. That emotional safety net interrupts the cascade of harmful physiological reactions, allowing the body's natural repair processes to function more effectively.

It's important to note that nurturing relationships require intention and effort. Deep connections don't happen by accident; they flourish in an environment of trust, empathy, and consistent communication. Quality always outweighs quantity here. A few truly meaningful relationships offer far more health benefits than numerous superficial ones. These bonds serve as a lifelong resource—a place for mutual support, laughter, and shared experiences that help maintain resilience.

Another key to deriving health benefits from relationships is reciprocity. Relationships that are one-sided, where effort or support feels imbalanced, can contribute to stress rather than alleviate it. Genuine give-and-take friendships and partnerships encourage a sense of purpose and belonging, both of which are linked to better mental health and lifespan. Giving support pushes us to look outward and cultivate compassion, while receiving care reminds us that we are valued and not alone in our struggles.

Technology has altered how we connect, and while digital communication offers incredible tools for staying in touch, it cannot fully replace face-to-face interaction. Physical presence enriches relationships by engaging multiple senses, fostering a deeper empathy and connection. Touch, eye contact, and shared physical experiences trigger the release of oxytocin—the so-called "bonding hormone"—which reduces anxiety and promotes feelings of safety. Whenever possible, prioritize in-person moments or even video calls over texting or social media to nurture genuine connection.

Supportive relationships extend beyond the personal sphere into the broader communal context. Being part of a community—a club, religious group, volunteer organization, or simply a circle of friends—enhances feelings of social integration and purpose. These communal ties create buffers against life's inevitable downturns and promote long-term adherence to healthy habits. For instance, community involvement often encourages physical activity, provides mental stimulation, and offers a network for advice or assistance when health challenges arise.

Moreover, relationships play an essential role in adopting and sustaining lifestyle changes aligned with longevity goals. A partner or friend who shares or supports your healthy eating habits, exercise routines, and stress management practices significantly increases the chances you'll stay committed. People are naturally influenced by those around them, so surrounding yourself with health-conscious individuals creates an environment where positive habits become the norm rather than the exception.

Emotional intimacy also correlates with better sleep quality, a critical but often overlooked component of lifespan extension. Being able to share thoughts and feelings without judgment helps reduce anxiety and calm the mind before bedtime. On the flip side, relationship conflicts or unresolved issues can disrupt sleep patterns, fueling a vicious cycle of stress and physical decline. So nurturing relationships is a crucial strategy for protecting the restorative power of sleep.

One practical approach to nurturing relationships for health is active listening—a skill that many underestimate but that profoundly strengthens bonds. When you listen attentively, without interrupting or planning your response, it validates the other person's experience and deepens mutual understanding. This, in turn, fosters trust and emotional safety, making it easier to navigate challenges together. Cultivating curiosity about others' perspectives and emotions encourages openness and strengthens connection.

It's equally important to recognize boundaries within relationships. Respecting personal space and allowing room for individual growth doesn't diminish closeness—in fact, it enhances it. Healthy relationships maintain a balance between togetherness and autonomy, offering support without smothering. When both parties feel free to be themselves, the relationship becomes a source of rejuvenation rather than stress.

Investing time in shared activities and rituals is another effective way to nourish relationships. Whether it's a weekly walk, cooking a meal together, or simply a regular phone call, these shared moments build memories and deepen connection. Such rituals become emotional anchors, providing stability and comfort across life's ups and downs. They serve as reminders that you're not alone, reinforcing your psychological and physical resilience.

Lifelong friendships and family ties also provide valuable health benefits by offering continuity and a sense of generational belonging. These long-term relationships weave a social fabric that supports identity, meaning, and purpose. Feeling connected to something bigger than oneself has been linked repeatedly to improved mental health and longevity. When challenged by illness or adversity, having a supportive network that spans years or even decades significantly improves recovery outcomes.

In short, nurturing relationships is not a luxury but a foundational pillar of longevity. Life's unpredictability becomes less daunting when met within a community that cares and supports. The physiological benefits alone—from reduced inflammation to enhanced immune function—justify dedicating energy toward building and maintaining meaningful social bonds. But there's a deeper truth at play: longevity is not just about living longer; it's about living richer. Relationships enrich our lives in ways that no supplement or technology can fully replicate.

Finally, consider that every interaction is an opportunity to strengthen your social connections. A smile, a kind word, an expression of gratitude—they all nurture the garden of relationships that sustains health and vitality. By approaching relationships with kindness, presence, and intention, you don't just improve your chances of a longer life—you enhance the quality of every moment along the way.

Chapter Twelve
ENVIRONMENTAL FACTORS AFFECTING LONGEVITY

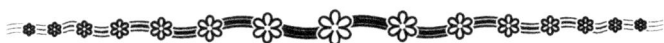

❈◦❈◦❈◦❈◦❈◦❈◦❈◦❈◦❈◦❈◦❈◦❈◦❈◦❈◦❈◦❈

The environments we live in shape our health in profound ways that often go unnoticed but carry immense influence over how long and well we live. From the air we breathe to the cleanliness of our living spaces, minimizing exposure to pollutants and toxins isn't just about avoiding illness—it's about actively preserving the body's natural defenses and reducing chronic stress on vital systems. Nature itself serves as a potent remedy; regular interaction with green spaces sparks measurable improvements in mood, inflammation, and even immune function. These environmental choices aren't passive circumstances but opportunities—small daily acts like improving indoor air quality or seeking out natural surroundings feed directly into the longevity equation. Recognizing that our surroundings can either nurture or erode our vitality empowers us to create living spaces that sustain health, offering one of the most accessible yet transformative avenues to extend both lifespan and the quality of years lived.

MINIMIZING EXPOSURE TO TOXINS

In the pursuit of a longer, healthier life, reducing the body's exposure to harmful toxins is a crucial and often overlooked element. Our environment is saturated with various chemicals and pollutants that quietly chip away at our well-being, accelerating aging and increasing the risk of chronic diseases. While we can't entirely escape every environmental insult, understanding how to minimize contact with these toxins empowers us to protect our bodies at a fundamental level.

Toxins are all around us—in the air we breathe, the food we eat, and the products we use daily. Some are obvious, like cigarette smoke or industrial pollutants, but many more go unnoticed because they're embedded in everyday items such as cleaning supplies, cosmetics, and even personal care products. These substances can disrupt the body's natural functions, impair cellular repair mechanisms, and lead to increased inflammation, which is a key driver of aging.

One of the most impactful moves you can make is re-evaluating the indoor environment where you spend the majority of your time. Indoor air often harbors volatile organic compounds (VOCs), mold spores, and dust that carry a cocktail of irritants and toxins. Investing in proper ventilation, using air purifiers with HEPA filters, and choosing natural or non-toxic cleaning products can drastically reduce your body's toxic burden. It's not about perfection but creating spaces that support your body's resilience instead of overwhelming it.

Food is another major vector for toxin exposure. Pesticides, herbicides, and heavy metals can find their way into our diet through conventionally grown produce and contaminated water sources. Opting for organic foods when possible, washing vegetables thoroughly, and favoring seasonal, locally sourced produce can significantly lower the intake of harmful chemicals. Remember, the food you eat not only fuels your day but also provides the raw materials your body uses to detoxify and regenerate at the cellular level.

In addition to careful food choices, being mindful about packaging and storage matters too. Many plastics contain endocrine-disrupting chemicals like BPA and phthalates, which can leach into food and beverages, especially when heated. Switching to glass, stainless steel, or BPA-free containers for food storage reduces this risk substantially. Even small changes like avoiding microwaving in plastic containers or sipping hot beverages from plastic cups contribute to long-term health benefits.

Personal care products often harbor hidden toxins that accumulate over time, including parabens, synthetic fragrances, and certain preservatives. These substances can interfere with hormones and promote oxidative stress—both harmful to longevity. One practical approach is scrutinizing labels and shifting toward products with transparent, natural ingredients. Better yet, fewer products overall mean fewer chemical exposures. Embracing simpler routines with natural oils or plant-based alternatives can be just as effective for cleansing and moisturizing, without the toxic load.

It's also vital to consider environmental toxins on a broader scale. Many urban areas have elevated levels of air pollution, which contributes to oxidative damage in the lungs and circulatory system. When living in or near high-pollution zones, strategies like wearing masks designed to filter particulates during peak traffic hours or engaging in outdoor activities when air quality is better can shield your respiratory system. Additionally, plants indoors not only beautify your space but help absorb toxins and refresh the air, creating a small personal oasis that supports health and longevity.

Occupational and lifestyle exposures are equally important. Jobs that involve handling chemicals, heavy metals, or prolonged exposure to dust and fumes require extra precautions such as protective gear and hygiene practices to limit toxic buildup. Even hobbies like painting or woodworking can introduce harmful substances, so dedicating a well-ventilated area for these activities and using masks or gloves goes a long way. The goal is to break the cycle of constant exposure so the body can focus its energy on healing and renewal rather than defense.

Another layer involves the water we drink and bathe in. Contaminants like chlorine, fluoride in high levels, heavy metals, and agricultural runoff can stealthily undermine health. Implementing water filtration systems that remove these pollutants helps ensure your cells are hydrated with clean, life-sustaining water. Clean water supports kidney function, digestion, and detoxification pathways, all fundamental to healthy aging.

Even seasonal and situational factors come into play. Wildfires, chemical spills, or pesticide spraying near residential areas can spike toxin levels unpredictably. Staying informed about local environmental alerts and having a plan to reduce exposure—such as closing windows, limiting outdoor activities, or using purifiers during these times—helps maintain a steady state of wellness. Proactivity and awareness create a protective buffer, reducing cumulative damage.

It's worth reflecting on why minimizing toxin exposure is so vital beyond just avoiding disease. Toxins provoke sustained immune activation, which drains resources and accelerates cellular aging. They cause DNA damage, impair mitochondrial function, and disturb hormone balance, creating a perfect storm that shortens both healthspan and lifespan. By consciously reducing the body's toxic load, you give it space to operate optimally, increasing not just years of life but the quality of those years.

Implementing these changes can seem daunting initially, but the process is a journey rather than a quick fix. Start small—perhaps swapping out just one toxic product or adding a plant to your living room. These incremental adjustments build momentum, creating an environment that nurtures vibrant health. The most sustainable change is one that fits seamlessly into daily life, becoming part of your identity rather than being a chore.

In the wider context of longevity, minimizing exposure to toxins is not an isolated task but integrates with nutrition, exercise, sleep, and mental well-being. When the body's internal and external environments are free from unnecessary chemical stressors, all these systems function more efficiently. Every breath you take, every meal you eat, and every product you apply is an opportunity to either support your body or challenge it.

Taking control of toxin exposure is an act of empowerment. It reframes longevity not as something that happens to you but as something you actively create. The choices you make about your surroundings send powerful messages to your cells, influencing gene expression and setting the stage for a vibrant, extended life. This isn't merely about avoiding harm—it's about crafting a life space that propels you toward your fullest potential.

Ultimately, the effort to minimize toxins aligns with a deeper respect for yourself and your environment. It acknowledges the intimate connection between what we put into our bodies, the spaces we occupy, and the future we envision. By stepping into this responsibility with intention, you reclaim control over one of the most critical determinants of aging and health. Your body deserves this care; your future self will thank you for it.

THE ROLE OF NATURE AND CLEAN LIVING SPACES

Living close to nature and maintaining clean, orderly environments can profoundly shape our path to longevity. The connection between our surroundings and how long and how well we live may sometimes be underestimated. But when you consider how the natural world influences stress reduction, air quality, physical activity, and even social interactions, it becomes clear that our environments function as more than just backdrops to our lives—they actively participate in our health outcomes.

Research consistently shows that exposure to natural settings—whether that's a forest, park, or even urban green spaces—correlates with lower levels of cortisol, the hormone linked to stress. Chronic stress has been tied to accelerated aging and a host of chronic conditions such as heart disease and cognitive decline. By contrast, regular contact with nature offers a natural reset button, helping to regulate stress hormones, improve mood, and promote feelings of well-being. Simply walking among trees or sitting near a body of water can trigger a cascade of physiological benefits, including lowered blood pressure and reduced inflammation, both critical matters when aiming to extend one's healthspan.

But it isn't just about proximity to large wilderness areas. The quality of our immediate living spaces plays an equally crucial role. A clean, toxin-free home environment is essential not only for comfort but for minimizing exposure to harmful chemicals and allergens. Everyday items like cleaning products, paints, and synthetic furnishings can emit volatile organic compounds (VOCs) that burden the respiratory system and disrupt hormonal balance. Over time, this invisible assault can wear down the body's defenses and reduce vitality. Households that prioritize cleanliness, decluttering, and the use of natural, non-toxic materials create sanctuaries that support healing and resilience on a cellular level.

Beyond chemical cleanliness, the organization of living spaces influences mental health in ways we often overlook. Clutter and disorder can increase anxiety and reduce the ability to focus, both of which drain cognitive reserves and leave us vulnerable to mental fatigue. On the other hand, a serene and orderly environment encourages mindfulness and relaxation, two essential components of longevity. People who intentionally design their spaces to foster calm and clarity are better equipped to manage daily stressors, ultimately protecting brain health over decades.

Nature and clean living spaces also encourage active lifestyles, which in turn promote longevity. When outdoor areas are accessible and inviting, physical activity becomes a natural part of daily routines—whether that's gardening, walking, or recreational sports. These activities not only improve cardiovascular health and muscular strength but also stimulate cognitive function through sensory engagement with the environment. Likewise, homes that provide uncluttered, well-lit areas encourage movement and reduce injury risk, helping older adults maintain independence longer.

Indoor air quality, often neglected, deserves attention too. Polluted air inside the home can come from cooking fumes, mold, dust mites, pet dander, and off-gassing from furniture or building materials. Poor indoor air quality has been linked to respiratory diseases and systemic inflammation, both of which undermine the body's ability to repair itself and stave off age-related decline. Investing in proper ventilation, air purifiers, and regular cleaning routines is a proven strategy to protect respiratory health and support longevity.

Interestingly, the benefits of nature exposure extend into social dimensions, which are vital for a long, happy life. Outdoor communal spaces provide the perfect backdrop for meaningful social interactions that strengthen support networks. Engaging with others in green environments tends to uplift mood, reduce feelings of isolation, and increase overall life satisfaction. Social engagement, combined with the calming effects of nature, creates a potent synergy that bolsters mental and emotional well-being—key drivers in the quest for extended lifespan.

Even the rhythmic patterns found in natural settings influence our internal biology. Natural light regulates circadian rhythms, which govern sleep-wake cycles, hormone release, and cellular repair processes. Living in environments that maximize exposure to natural daylight—and minimize disruptive artificial lighting in the evening—helps maintain these rhythms. This alignment supports restorative sleep, which is foundational to longevity, as it enables the body to heal and rejuvenate itself each night.

The design of living spaces, both indoors and outdoors, can further amplify these benefits. Incorporating natural elements such as plants, water features, and natural materials brings aspects of the outside world inside, creating a soothing ambiance that reduces stress and fosters concentration. Biophilic design isn't just a trendy concept; it taps into deeply rooted human needs for nature connection, which, when met, improves physiological and psychological resilience.

For individuals committed to longevity, understanding the impact of environmental quality should prompt actionable change. This might mean advocating for greener neighborhoods, integrating more natural elements into home decor, or adopting cleaning habits that avoid toxins. Each step taken to harmonize with nature and cultivate clean, restorative living spaces enhances the body's capacity to withstand the effects of aging.

Ultimately, longevity isn't achieved through isolated decisions but through the ongoing optimization of the many environmental factors that surround us. The air we breathe, the light we soak in, the surfaces we touch, and the communities we engage with all weave together to influence how long and how well we live. Prioritizing time spent in nature and keeping our living environments clean and nurturing awakens a vital layer of support for the body's natural defenses and repair mechanisms.

Incorporating these practices also aligns with lifelong health in a deeply sustainable way. Unlike quick fixes or supplement routines, engaging with nature and fostering clean living spaces create daily habits that rejuvenate both mind and body. This holistic approach strengthens your foundation for longevity, offering a shield against the wear and tear that accumulates over time.

As we continue exploring environmental influences on lifespan, keep in mind that your surroundings are not passive—they're active participants in your health journey. By embracing nature and cultivating spaces that promote purity and peace, you're investing in the most essential and long-lasting asset: yourself.

Chapter Thirteen
CREATING YOUR PERSONALIZED LONGEVITY PLAN

=•=❄=❄=❄=❄=❄==❄==❄==❄==❄=❄=❄=❄=•=

Crafting a longevity plan that fits your unique life starts with a clear-eyed assessment of where you stand today—your health markers, habits, and environment—and then pairing that insight with goals that inspire real change, not just temporary fixes. This plan isn't about chasing the latest fad but about weaving together sustainable actions that match your rhythms and values, helping you build momentum one step at a time. You'll draw from proven strategies, yes, but tailor them so they feel manageable and meaningful, making longevity a natural extension of your daily choices rather than a distant ideal. The real power lies in customizing a path that respects your individuality while pushing toward greater vitality, so each day becomes a deliberate investment in a longer, fuller life.

ASSESSING YOUR CURRENT HEALTH PROFILE

Before diving into actionable steps that can lengthen your lifespan and elevate your wellbeing, it's vital to take an honest, comprehensive look at your current health status. This self-assessment forms the foundation of any personalized longevity plan. You can't steer a ship without first knowing your coordinates; similarly, understanding your health profile is essential to chart a clear course toward better health and extended years.

Assessment is more than just ticking off boxes during your annual checkup. It's about gathering meaningful data points that illuminate how your body and mind are functioning today—and identifying which areas demand the most attention. You may already have a general sense of your health, but without thorough evaluation, you risk overlooking hidden issues that could undermine your longevity efforts down the road.

Begin with a detailed health history review. This means going beyond the surface, asking yourself about chronic conditions, recurring symptoms, family medical background, medications, and lifestyle habits. This overview acts as a roadmap, revealing patterns that may increase your risk for age-related diseases or functional decline. Family history, for instance, often provides critical clues to genetic predispositions, while lifestyle choices offer insight into modifiable factors you can target right away.

Equally important is understanding your body's current metabolic and physiological status. Basic measurements such as blood pressure, resting heart rate, body mass index (BMI), and waist circumference offer revealing information. Elevated blood pressure or excess abdominal fat often serve as red flags for cardiovascular risk or metabolic syndrome, conditions linked to lower life expectancy. Tracking these metrics over time helps gauge progress and guides adjustments within your longevity plan.

Laboratory testing is an invaluable tool to uncover subtle imbalances or risks invisible to the naked eye. Comprehensive blood panels can measure cholesterol levels, blood sugar, inflammation markers, and nutrient deficiencies—all of which profoundly influence aging and healthspan. For example, elevated markers of inflammation often predict chronic disease development, while anemia or vitamin D deficiency can silently sap energy and immune defense. Your goal in assessing these labs isn't simply to know the numbers, but to understand their context and implications for your unique biology.

Equally vital is gauging your functional fitness and physical capabilities. Longevity does not mean just adding years; it means maximizing vitality in those years. How easily do you perform daily activities? Can you climb stairs without breathlessness or maintain balance to prevent falls? Assessing mobility, strength, and endurance highlights your current physical resilience and points to areas needing reinforcement. Functional capacity measurements often reveal risks that traditional biomarkers can miss, such as early sarcopenia (muscle loss) or gait instability—both predictors of premature frailty.

Mental and cognitive health assessment must be a core part of your evaluation. Brain health forms a critical strand in the longevity tapestry. Simple screening tools and questionnaires can reveal signs of mood disorders, memory challenges, or cognitive decline, which often precede more serious neurodegenerative diseases. Keeping track of your mental wellbeing and identifying stressors or psychiatric symptoms opens doors to early interventions that protect your mind as well as your body.

Sleep quality and patterns are frequently overlooked in general health assessments, yet they are indispensable components of longevity. Sleep deprivation or fragmented sleep disrupts hormonal balance, immunity, brain function, and cellular repair—all essential for healthy aging. Self-reported sleep diaries, wearable tracking devices, or professional sleep studies, if necessary, provide insight into how restorative your nightly rest truly is. Learning where your sleep falters enables targeted strategies to improve recovery and resilience.

In recent years, genetic testing has emerged as a powerful adjunct to traditional health profiling. Understanding your genetic predispositions lets you tailor lifestyle adjustments to counter inherited risks or enhance protective traits. While genes don't write your destiny, they frame a set of probabilities that smart lifestyle choices can meaningfully influence. Consulting with healthcare professionals trained in genetics can help interpret this data responsibly, avoiding alarmism while maximizing benefit.

Beyond the quantifiable, don't neglect environmental and social factors that shape your health. Your living conditions, exposure to toxins, stress levels, and quality of interpersonal relationships cast a long shadow on longevity outcomes. Assessing these elements helps ensure your plan encompasses not only biology but the wider ecosystem in which you live, work, and thrive. You might discover, for instance, that reducing exposure to urban pollution or cultivating stronger social ties could be as impactful as dietary changes or exercise.

One more critical dimension to appraise is your current health literacy and readiness for change. Longevity becomes achievable only when motivation, knowledge, and support align. Being honest about what you know, what you're willing to try, and the barriers you face sets realistic expectations for how you'll build sustainable habits. Reflection and goal-setting exercise at this stage make the roadmap personal and actionable, avoiding generic advice that fails to resonate with your lifestyle.

Successfully assessing your current health profile requires a combination of self-inquiry, clinical evaluation, and sometimes specialized testing. This holistic approach uncovers subtle clues, strengthens understanding, and spotlights priority areas ripe for intervention. It also empowers you to track progress objectively, turning longevity ambitions into measurable milestones.

Ultimately, a thorough, honest health assessment isn't a one-time event, but the ongoing pulse check of your longevity journey. Reassessing periodically ensures your personalized plan remains aligned with evolving needs and goals. Health isn't static; it fluctuates with time, experiences, and choices. Being attuned to these shifts allows you to course-correct and sustain progress over decades rather than months.

As you move forward, remember that the power to extend your healthspan begins with knowledge—knowledge rooted in an accurate, nuanced picture of your current state. Once you've completed this crucial step, you'll be positioned to create a longevity plan that's not only scientifically grounded but also uniquely yours. It's the essential first stride on any path to living vibrantly longer and better.

BUILDING SUSTAINABLE AND EFFECTIVE HABITS

Creating a personalized longevity plan is more than gathering facts or trying out the latest health craze—it's about making lasting changes that truly fit your lifestyle. When you think about extending your healthspan, the habits you build daily hold the key. Without consistency and sustainability, even the most scientifically grounded approaches won't yield the results you want. That's why this part of your longevity journey focuses on how to develop effective habits that endure, not just quick fixes or temporary enthusiasm.

Habits form the backbone of any successful longevity strategy because they shape your behavior over time, becoming almost automatic. The science of habit formation tells us that repetition creates neural pathways that make certain actions feel natural and effortless. But just as habits can build you up, they can also tear your progress down if they're not aligned with your goals. It's essential to identify which habits support your vitality and which ones stand in the way. This means making deliberate choices about where you spend your energy on a daily basis and how those actions contribute to your overall well-being.

One of the most important principles in building sustainable habits is starting small. Large, sweeping changes might be exhilarating, but they're rarely maintainable. Consider how a tiny habit—like drinking a glass of water each morning or walking for five minutes after lunch—can serve as the foundation for bigger transformations. Those small steps are easier to incorporate and less intimidating, which lowers resistance. Gradually, as new behaviors become routine, you can scale up the intensity or frequency without burning out. This approach respects both your biology and psychology, giving your brain time to adapt and your motivation to stay intact.

Another crucial factor is aligning habits with your personal values and lifestyle. When habits resonate with what matters most to you, they spark intrinsic motivation, making it far more likely you'll stick with them in the long run. For example, if you cherish time with family, incorporating a daily walk with a loved one can simultaneously bolster your social connections and physical health. When habits feel personally meaningful, they shift from being chores to purposeful actions. Additionally, tailoring habits to your daily rhythm—whether you're an early riser or a night owl—helps avoid unnecessary friction that often leads to abandonment of new routines.

Accountability also plays a pivotal role. Sharing your intentions with a supportive community or accountability partner creates an external structure that reinforces your commitment. Humans are social creatures wired for connection, and tapping into that can provide the nudge you need on days when motivation lags. Whether it's a workout buddy, a group challenge, or simply reporting your progress to a friend, external accountability leverages social dynamics that boost habit adherence. But even without a partner, self-monitoring—such as journaling or tracking your progress digitally—helps maintain awareness and correct course when necessary.

It's easy to underestimate how much your environment influences your habits as well. We are creatures of habit partly because environments cue behaviors, often below conscious awareness. If your kitchen counters are cluttered with tempting snacks, trying to maintain a healthy diet becomes a daily uphill battle. But if you rearrange those counters so that fresh fruits and vegetables are front and center, making nutritious choices happens almost by default. The same applies to exercise gear, sleep environment, or even the timing of your activities. Control your surroundings to make the right behaviors the safe, simple, and natural options.

One pattern you'll want to avoid is relying solely on willpower. While determination is useful in short bursts, it's a limited resource that depletes quickly under stress. Habits, by contrast, operate with less conscious effort and help conserve willpower for moments when it truly matters. By automating healthy behaviors, you transform decision fatigue into steadiness. That's why designing systems that support your habits—like meal prepping to avoid unhealthy choices or scheduling exercise sessions at the same time each day—can keep you on track even when motivation dips.

Expect setbacks. They are an inevitable part of the process, not a sign of failure. What defines successful habit formation is resilience—the ability to get back on course after a stumble. This perspective keeps you grounded and reduces the all-or-nothing mindset that often sabotages progress. Instead of seeing a missed workout or one unhealthy meal as a catastrophe, regard it as data. Why did it happen? What barriers got in the way? How can you better prepare to handle these challenges next time? That kind of self-compassion leads not just to sustainability but to deep and lasting change.

The key to integrating new habits is to weave them into the fabric of your existing routines. This technique, called habit stacking, pairs a new behavior with an established one. If you always brush your teeth in the morning, try adding a minute of deep breathing right afterward. Or if you take a coffee break every afternoon, use a few of those minutes to do light stretches or mindfulness exercises. Habit stacking leverages the natural flow of your day, turning what could be a struggle into a seamless and automatic part of life. Over time, a chain of small, positive habits can multiply to create a powerful foundation for longevity.

Intrinsic motivation often waxes and wanes, so developing a vision that keeps you inspired is invaluable. Rather than focusing only on "not getting sick" or "living longer," consider the quality of life you want to enjoy. Visualize yourself engaging fully in the activities you love, interacting vibrantly with friends and family, or pursuing passions with energy. This vision fuels your commitment and transforms health behaviors into expressions of the life you choose, not just obligations. That internal narrative becomes a compass guiding each decision and habit you cultivate.

Technology offers another useful ally in habit formation. Apps for tracking nutrition, exercise, sleep, or meditation can provide timely reminders and insight into patterns that might escape notice. Simple feedback loops make your progress visible, enhancing motivation, and empowering you to adjust routines before small issues turn into big problems. But be cautious not to become overly dependent on screens or metrics. The goal is to develop habits so ingrained they persist naturally, with technology serving as a helpful guide, not a crutch.

Ultimately, building habits that support longevity is a journey of transformation, where each small, sustainable step compounds over time. You're not chasing perfection; you're cultivating a lifestyle that aligns with your deepest values and supports a vibrant, extended life. Once the habits take root, they become the engine driving your health and well-being forward, giving you the freedom to embrace life fully. This process requires patience but rewards with a vitality that can extend decades beyond what you might assume today.

Remember, the secret to longevity is less about radical change and more about steady, consistent progress. Sustainable, effective habits form the foundation of this progress, making longevity an achievable and inspiring goal. By investing in the habits that nourish your body, mind, and spirit, you'll create a personalized plan that not only extends your years but enriches every moment within them.

EMBRACING A VIBRANT, LONGER LIFE

As we reach the culmination of this journey through the science and practice of longevity, it's clear that living longer doesn't simply mean adding years to your life — it means adding life to your years. Embracing a vibrant, extended lifespan is not about chasing perfection or waiting for miraculous breakthroughs. Instead, it's a deliberate choice to weave together evidence-based habits that elevate the quality of every day we have. It's about seeing longevity as a grand, ongoing project that involves your mind, body, and community in a harmonious balance.

Longevity is often misunderstood as an elusive, distant goal reserved for the few who are genetically blessed or have access to cutting-edge clinics. Yet, the truth is far more empowering: while genetics set the stage, your daily actions and environments play starring roles in how you age. What you eat, how you move, the way you manage stress, the quality of your sleep, your social ties, and even how you nurture your mental resilience—all of these pieces create the mosaic of your healthspan. It's this comprehensive, interconnected approach, more than anything else, that paves the path to a vibrant, longer life.

One of the most inspiring realizations is the body's remarkable capacity to adapt and improve throughout life. The science of epigenetics reveals that genes don't rigidly dictate our fate. Instead, lifestyle choices can switch genetic expression toward greater health and vitality. This means that regardless of your starting point, adopting practical strategies around nutrition, exercise, and holistic self-care — even in midlife or beyond — can profoundly influence how you age. The key is consistency and willingness to evolve your habits as you learn and grow.

Longevity isn't a checklist filled out once and forgotten. It's a daily practice, refined over time. It's about shifting from reactive health care—waiting to be ill then treating symptoms—to proactive, preventive care that sustains and enhances function. You don't have to overhaul your life overnight; small, deliberate changes accumulate and compound in ways that can surprise you. Filling your plate with anti-inflammatory foods, engaging in physical activity that you enjoy, carving out time to rest and rejuvenate, and fostering meaningful relationships are all accessible, impactful steps.

Equally important is the mindset you bring to this endeavor. Aging can be viewed not as decline but as an opportunity—a chance to savor wisdom, cultivate purpose, and deepen connections. When you embrace longevity with curiosity and optimism, rather than fear or resistance, it transforms how you perceive your body and your future. This shift in perspective fuels motivation, helping you sustain the lifestyle choices that support a longer, fuller life. What you believe about aging matters just as much as what you do.

At the heart of embracing a vibrant, longer life is the recognition that health is multidimensional. Physical vitality and cognitive sharpness are intertwined with emotional well-being and social engagement. Longevity science increasingly underscores that isolation and chronic stress detract from lifespan as much as poor diet or inactivity. Conversely, communities rich in connection and support elevate resilience and longevity. Investing in relationships, nurturing empathy, and fostering a sense of belonging bring profound health dividends that often go unmeasured yet are deeply felt.

You've also seen how modern longevity science doesn't dismiss time-honored wisdom but rather blends it with innovative research and technology. This synergy opens exciting possibilities for personalized health plans tuned to your unique genetic makeup, lifestyle preferences, and evolving health metrics. It's not about chasing every new trend or expensive therapy; it's about integrating proven, sustainable practices that enhance your body's natural ability to heal and adapt.

In many ways, embracing a longer life is an act of hope and responsibility—hope that science and human spirit will continue to advance, and responsibility to care for yourself as the precious resource you are. It means crafting a vision of aging where vitality, purpose, and happiness persist alongside physical health. When we take this holistic approach, longevity becomes less about numbers on a calendar and more about the quality of experiences, the richness of relationships, and the joy found in daily living.

As you reflect on your own journey, remember that this is an ongoing path with many seasons. Life will inevitably present challenges, from unexpected health setbacks to emotional upheavals. Yet the practices you develop empower you to navigate those ups and downs with greater resilience and grace. Longevity isn't about perfection; it's about persistence and adaptability. It's about thriving in the face of change and continuously seeking ways to nurture your well-being.

Your longer life can also be one filled with adventure and learning, a canvas on which to paint new goals and dreams. Aging with vibrancy means maintaining curiosity about the world and yourself. It encourages exploring fresh activities, embracing new mindsets, and finding joy in simple pleasures. The journey toward longevity is not only scientific and structured but richly human and deeply personal.

What stands out most clearly at the end of this exploration is that true longevity blossoms when your lifestyle aligns with your values. Pursuing practices solely out of a fear of death or decline is exhausting and unsustainable. But when your daily choices resonate with what gives your life meaning—whether family, creativity, service, or connection—you find the motivation to uphold these healthy habits over the long haul. Longevity then becomes a natural extension of how fully you live each moment, a testament to your commitment to yourself and those you love.

In summation, embracing a vibrant, longer life is a multifaceted commitment. It's about harnessing science, cultivating support systems, and fostering an optimistic, resilient mindset. It invites you to view aging not as a limitation but a dynamic chapter filled with promise and potential. The strategies detailed throughout this book are the tools—your foundation for creating a life marked by energy, clarity, and fulfillment well into your later years.

Ultimately, the choice is yours to make. You have both the power and the opportunity to shape your healthspan—transforming the timeline of your life into a tale of vitality and purpose. This journey calls for courage, curiosity, and consistent care. Step forward with confidence knowing that the vibrant, longer life you envision is within reach, built day by day through the habits you embrace and the spirit you nurture.

APPENDIX A
RESOURCES
AND TOOLS FOR
LONGEVITY SUCCESS

As you embark on the journey toward a longer, healthier life, having the right resources and tools at your disposal can make all the difference. This section gathers practical guides, reliable sources, and effective tools designed to empower you in applying the longevity principles explored throughout this book. The goal is simple: give you a solid foundation to make informed choices and build habits that last.

First, when it comes to trustworthy information, lean on scientific journals and evidence-based health websites. Subscribing to newsletters from reputable institutions focused on aging research will keep you updated on breakthroughs and best practices. These platforms often distill complex studies into actionable insights, sparing you from misinformation or hype.

Tracking your progress is an indispensable part of any longevity plan. Tools like wearable fitness trackers help monitor your daily activity, heart rate variability, and sleep patterns. They provide immediate feedback, making it easier to fine-tune exercise routines and rest cycles—two pillars for maximizing lifespan. Pair these devices with mobile apps tailored to nutritional tracking or meditation, and you create a comprehensive system for self-awareness and adjustment.

Another key asset is genetic testing services that offer insight into your unique biological makeup. While genetics don't dictate destiny, knowing your predispositions allows you to personalize lifestyle choices—from diet preferences to stress management tactics—more effectively. Consider combining this information with professional guidance to avoid misinterpretation and to build a targeted approach.

Don't underestimate the power of community. Longevity thrives not only through physical and mental practices but also through social engagement. Online forums and in-person groups focused on health, nutrition, or mindful aging provide motivation, accountability, and new perspectives. Sharing successes and challenges can keep you motivated beyond the initial excitement.

Books, podcasts, and online courses from experts who bring clarity to the science of aging will continue to inspire and educate. They allow you to stay curious, adapt to emerging knowledge, and deepen your understanding without getting overwhelmed.

Finally, embrace tools that promote balance and recovery: guided mindfulness apps, blue-light filtering glasses to protect your sleep cycle, and devices that encourage regular movement even during busy workdays. Longevity is a delicate balance between pushing forward and honoring rest.

In essence, this toolkit is about equipping you with what you need to build resilience, foster habits that support vital health, and stay engaged in a lifelong quest for well-being. Implement these resources thoughtfully, listen to your body's signals, and adjust your strategies as you grow. With the right tools in hand, the vision of a vibrant, extended life becomes not just attainable but sustainable.

www.ingramcontent.com/pod-product-compliance
Lightning Source LLC
Chambersburg PA
CBHW031202270326
41931CB00006B/365